The Spinal Cord Injury Handbook for Patients and Their Families

Richard C. Senelick, MD,
with Karla Dougherty

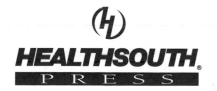

HEALTHSOUTH
P R E S S

This book is not intended to replace personal medical care and/or professional supervision; there is no substitute for the experience and information that your doctor or health professional can provide. Rather, it is our hope that this book will provide additional information to help people understand the nature of spinal cord injury and its effects on its survivors and their families.

Proper treatment should always be tailored to the individual. If you read something in this book that seems to conflict with any of your doctors' or health professionals' instructions, contact them. There may be sound reasons for recommending treatment that may differ from the information presented in this book.

If you have any questions about any treatment in this book, please consult your doctor or healthcare professional.

Also, the names and cases used in this book do not represent actual people, but are composite cases drawn from several sources.

© 1998 by HealthSouth Press
One HealthSouth Parkway, Birmingham, Alabama 35243

Published by HealthSouth Press

Library of Congress Catalog Card Number: 98-73410
ISBN: 1-891525-01-8
First HealthSouth Printing
10 9 8 7 6 5 4 3 2 1
HealthSouth Press and colophon are registered trademarks of HealthSouth

Printed in the United States of America

Dedication

This book is dedicated to the patients and their families who have not only survived spinal cord injury but who have triumphed. To these men and women who have learned to move past seemingly insurmountable obstacles to live lives that are different, but no less accomplished and fulfilling.

Through them, we have learned so much, both intellectually and emotionally. We have seen first hand the resiliency and adaptability of the human spirit, the day-to-day strength and resolve, that our spinal cord injury rehabilitation patients and their families continue to show us — and the world.

The Facts About HealthSouth

HealthSouth Corporation is the nation's largest physical rehabilitation healthcare provider with over 75,000 patients being treated in its facilities every day.

The HealthSouth network includes rehabilitation hospitals and acute-care medical centers, as well as outpatient rehabilitation, ambulatory surgery, and diagnostic imaging centers. Some of its diverse services include the treatment of spinal cord injury, sports injuries, brain injury, stroke, pain management, oncology rehabilitation, geriatric rehabilitation, and such diagnostic services as mammography, magnetic resonance imaging (MRI), nuclear medicine, and ultrasound.

HealthSouth Press has been created to help patients and their families understand the ramifications of their injury or illness. All of its books are created to help families learn how to cope with life's unexpected changes. And, above all, each book is designed to show, in compassionate and intelligent terms, that you, the reader, are not alone.

Acknowledgments

We would like to thank Tony Tanner, Executive Vice President of HealthSouth, for his support and leadership in the creation of the HealthSouth Press. We would also like to thank our other Editorial Board members for their help: Leslie Scrushy, and Kathryn Hughes. Thanks, too, to Gerald Nix, Amy Corcoran, and Laura Fredericks of HealthSouth for their help in seeing this manuscript through to fruition, as well as the entire production and art staff of HealthSouth Press.

We would also like to thank John Sikora, Nancy Lewis, CRRN, and Dr. Gilbert Brenes at HealthSouth Harmarville Rehabilitation Hospital for their help and guidance in ensuring the accuracy of this book. Further, Selena Morgan, Mari Feist, and Sara Dwyer from the HealthSouth Rehabilitation Institute of San Antonio Departments of Physical Therapy and Occupational Therapy were also invaluable in keeping this book timely and accurate. We thank them for their help in educating patients, families, and ourselves about the effects of spinal cord injury. Without them, and all the other members of the HealthSouth rehabilitation team, we cannot imagine how we would be able to care for the patients and their families.

CONTENTS

A BRAVE NEW WORLD

- *It was one of those special summer days when the sun starts shining early in the morning, the breezes are cool and soothing, the clouds glide through the blue, blue sky, and nobody within a 60-mile radius feels like working. The people in Ray's office were no exception. Since they'd all spent the last week working long hours to get caught up with the inventory, the boss decided to let everybody off early. With a whoop and a holler, Ray and his pals jumped into his pickup and raced to the local gravel pit that had recently been turned into a lake. They couldn't wait to take a dip in the cool, clear water and float on their backs, the sun on their faces. It took only seconds for Ray to strip down to his trunks, race to a ledge 6 feet above the water, and dive headfirst into the shimmering water below. A beat. Two seconds. One minute passed. Five minutes. Where was Ray? He hadn't surfaced. His friends swam out to the spot where Ray had disappeared and then dragged his limp body out and up the side of the lake. He was unconscious; his head had struck a large rock unseen from above. He had what we call a fracture to the C5 vertebra. Ray couldn't move his arms or legs; he had broken his neck. Within a week, thanks to emergency room care and successful neurosurgery, Ray could feel a tingle in his arms; he could shrug his shoulders and move his upper arms. But he would need months of rehabilitation — and would use a wheelchair for the rest of his life. If only he had remembered the diver's rule: "Feet first, first time."*

- *It was an incident that played over and over again in Betty's mind. She had been working late, trying to meet a deadline, one stormy New England night. She was the last one to leave the office and the snow had begun to fall in clusters; she could barely see her car in the deserted parking lot. Betty almost slipped as she walked over hidden icy patches, but she somehow managed to get behind the wheel, the wipers on, and the heat going full steam. She slowly, slowly drove her car out of the lot; she wasn't a reckless driver and she wasn't going to rush anywhere in this storm. But conditions worsened. The storm had turned into a blizzard, complete with icy wind, swirling snow, and piling drifts. Suddenly, without warning, Betty hit a patch of ice on the highway and lost control of the car. It spun to the side and hit a cement barrier head-on. Crash! Betty felt as if a load of bricks had hit her chest and back; she struggled to breathe. When an EMS crew arrived and carried her from the car, Betty realized she couldn't move her legs; she couldn't feel them. An X-ray subsequently revealed a burst fracture in her lumbar region at the L1 vertebra. The result? A loss of bladder and bowel control and the use of her legs. Although surgery removed the bony fragments that had strangled these nerves, Betty needed rehabilitation. Over time, she learned to walk again with braces, but she would always have problems controlling her bowels and bladder. Yet Betty felt lucky. She had survived a terrible storm — and she was alive.*

- *The holidays were always a good time to find part-time work, to get a little extra cash for Christmas presents. Janie sure could use some money; her kids had their hearts set on the newest toys advertised on TV, and she didn't want to have to tell them no. When a good friend asked Janie to help with her cleaning service, she jumped at it. Without a high school degree or special training, Janie's opportunities were limited. One of the first jobs they had was a tough one: They had to scrape paint and soot off the windows of a three-story house. Janie went about her chores with her usual grit and determination. Thoughts of all the wonderful presents she'd be able to get her children danced in her head as she cleaned. She was up in the attic scraping the last bit of paint off the last window in the house when it happened. She took a step and her foot broke through the old wood floor. She fell over 12 feet, swooping down like a clipped bird, through the floor to the high-ceilinged living room below. Before she even had time to scream she had landed flat on her back on the oak parquet floor. Stunned, in shock, unable to move, Janie howled in pain. Within hours, she heard the news: She had dislocated her T5 vertebra, which literally pressed her spinal cord flat. Janie was now numb from her breasts down; her legs were paralyzed. She was still able to get her kids their Christmas presents except for the one they wanted more than anything else in the world: their mom like she was before.*

- *The determined face of Christopher Reeve, appearing on our TV screens and magazine covers, is a familiar one. We all feel we know this strikingly handsome, talented actor, who, in the prime of his career and his life, was cut down in a heartbeat while jumping a horse over a fence. One second he had had it all. The next, he was lying on the ground, gasping for breath, gasping for life. The fracture at the very top of his neck not only cut the nerves that controlled his arms and legs but also took away the nerves and muscles which allowed him to breathe. Christopher Reeve can no longer take a breath on his own or live without the small machine strapped to the back of his wheelchair. A high quadriplegic, he speaks for the almost 400,000 people who suffer from spinal cord injury in America today. He speaks for all of us in his appeal not to give up, not to despair, that life lived differently is still life.*

Hopping. Skipping. Dancing. Jumping. Walking. Putting one foot in front of the other. Taking a breath of fresh, clean air. We take these things for granted. And we should. But when we lose these basic human functions, these abilities that many equate with youth, vigor, and being alive, we lose so much more: a universal belief in what we consider a full, rich life.

Ask Christopher Reeve. Or Janie, Ray, or Betty. They can tell you what they had to learn, what they had to fight, what extraordinary stress they had to deal with. They can tell you all this — and more. They can tell you how they survived.

THE SPINAL CORD INJURY HANDBOOK
FOR PATIENTS AND THEIR FAMILIES

In these pages, you will learn exactly what these survival skills entail as well as the nuts and bolts of spinal cord injury (SCI). You'll discover exactly what spinal cord injury is and what to expect when specific vertebrae are injured at specific regions along your spinal column. You'll find out the complications that can arise from spinal cord injury, from pressure sores and osteoporosis to such injury-specific conditions as autonomic dysreflexia and muscle shortening, or contractures. You'll also learn how to cope with the problems at the core of SCI: mobility, bowel and bladder control, sexual dysfunction, and depression. And, most important of all, you'll learn how rehabilitation works and how you, a family member or survivor, can help ensure its success.

In short, like those people you have just met in our examples, you — and your loved one — will learn how to live, and live well, in a new life.

SPINAL CORD INJURY IS UNIQUE

The people you've met in this introduction are only words on paper. Even Christopher Reeve is no closer to you than your television set or movie screen. They are abstract. Think instead of your *own* spinal cord injury or the spinal cord injury survivor in *your* life. The element that shouts out, that hits with a profound jolt, is the fact that in moments, your entire being is changed. Suddenly, you are unable to move when, moments before, you had been riding a horse, the wind in your hair; doing figure eights on the ice; or driving along in your car, the radio full blast.

The physical consequences of spinal cord injury are very basic: A specific section of your spinal column is injured, causing a specific malfunction. If the injury occurred to the lumbar or thoracic sections of your spinal column (the L or T sections that affected Janie and Betty), you may lose control of your bladder and bowels. Your lower limbs will be affected and your condition will be called paraplegia. If the injury occurred further up the spinal cord, the cervical and upper regions of the thoracic sections (the C or T sections), your condition would be considered quadriplegia, or, as it is called today, tetraplegia. You would not only suffer the same losses as a paraplegic, but, like Ray, your body would take more slings. Your arms and your legs would be paralyzed; you would lose bowel and bladder control. And, as with Christopher Reeve, you might not be able to breathe without a ventilator.

But, as universal and predictable as the physical ramifications of spinal cord injury are, the mind colors everything and makes your injury unique: *your* individual reactions, *your* feelings, *your* fears, and *your* hopes.

Because along with the sudden, traumatic change in your body, in your ability to dance, jump, dash, and walk, comes this profound irony: Your mind is intact. You know exactly what happened to you. You know that you cannot move. That you cannot control your bladder or bowels. That the normal, everyday tasks of daily living are most likely altered.

More irony: The 7,800 spinal cord injuries that occur each year usually happen to strong, vibrant young men and women involved in sports, adventure vacations, driving accidents, or falls. They literally lose their path in life before they've taken many steps. They come to realize that the life they'd chosen, the one they took for granted, the one that moved in predictable ways, would never be the same.

It makes sense that this situation can result in depression — and desperation — as you seek unreliable "cures," as you hold on to unrealistic hope.

To keep depression at bay, to keep their strong dreams and desires alive, many people cling to hope, any hope, no matter how desperate, expensive, or ultimately detrimental to successful rehabilitation it can be.

But hope does not have to have this desperate edge. As you will learn throughout this book, there is realistic hope and very real progress that can be made, especially with the right rehabilitation.

More and more research is coming out every day about new treatments, new diagnoses, and new avenues of rehabilitation. Although a cure is far in the future, *The New York Times* reports that there have been successful experiments in regeneration of spinal nerves. New advances in medication suggest that we might be able to coax our spinal nerves to mend themselves. We also know that there is a very potent window of opportunity within the first 12 hours of injury. If the spinal cord is not severed completely, steroids can help restore some movement if given quickly enough in an acute-care hospital.

In the meantime, the most powerful tool you can have in coping with spinal cord injury is education. Read this book. Use it. Learn the newest diagnostic tools available. Discover the most successful rehabilitation treatments. Find out what you can do to keep progress going and motivation high.

With education comes acceptance. And, armed with acceptance, you can come to the realization that life is not over. You have just taken a different path.

There are still opportunities, new goals, to greet you every day. Some doors may have closed, but at the same time, others have put out their welcome mat. This happened to Ray, Betty, Janie — and Christopher Reeve, who not only received a standing ovation at the 1997 Academy Awards, but who also recently directed his first movie to critical acclaim.

Let us begin our journey to your new life. It's time to get yourself — and the people you love — back.

CHAPTER ONE

WHAT SPINAL CORD INJURY IS — AND ISN'T

"The occasion is piled high with difficulty, and we must rise with the occasion. As our case is new, so we must think anew and act anew."

– Abraham Lincoln
Annual message to Congress, 1862

Bart had spent all day fixing the tiles on his roof. It had been a difficult job: The sun had been beating down on his head, and the loose tiles seemed to be in the farthest nooks and crannies of the dormers. But, at last, he was done. His roof held fast. "Let it rain now!" he shouted to the sky with satisfaction. He had done a backbreaking job and he was proud of it.

Wiping the sweat off his forehead, Bart started down his ladder. He held on to the side with one arm; the other held his pail of supplies. Just as his feet were in the rungs, the wind picked up. A cloth he'd used and neglected to pick up blew into his face. Startled, Bart automatically swiped at his eyes. He lost his balance. The ladder wobbled. The pail dropped with a clatter on the ground. Bart screamed as he fell three stories to his driveway, the ladder landing with a thud on top of him.

The unthinkable had happened. In seconds, Bart's world had changed dramatically. When he was rushed to the hospital, he learned that the nerves that made up his spinal cord in the lower region were destroyed. He would never be able to climb a ladder again. Bart would have to learn to live without the use of his legs.

One of the characteristics of any injury, any traumatic accident, is its suddenness, its cruel twisting of a fate that seemed so certain only moments ago. But spinal cord injury is unique in its predictability. When a certain area of the spinal cord is damaged or destroyed, it will affect certain bodily functions. Period. "A" equals "B."

SPINAL CORDS

Some vital statistics:
- *There are between 250,000 and 400,000 people with spinal cord injuries living in the United States today.*
- *Most spinal cord injuries are caused in motor vehicle driving accidents (44%).*
- *The next most common arena for SCI is violence (24%), followed closely by accidental falls (22%).*
- *Those with the most risk? It's usually a male (82%) between 16 and 30 years of age. He will most likely be single (53%) and may or may not be employed. He may be a student.*

- Damage in the high cervical segments of the neck area will affect breathing, the neck, arm, and leg muscles.
- Damage in the thoracic segments of the trunk will affect the trunk and legs.
- Damage in the lumbar and sacral segments in the lower back will affect the legs.
- And damage in any of these areas can affect bowel, bladder, and sexual function.

Because spinal cord injury is so "cut and dried," a basic knowledge of the nervous system and the spinal column will help immeasurably in understanding your problems.

ANATOMY 101: THE NERVOUS SYSTEM

The spinal cord is the largest nerve in your body. Think of it as a thick telephone cable, one that connects the brain to other parts of your body. Both your brain and your spinal cord make up the central nervous system (CNS) — the AT&T of your body. Together, they make sure that what you see or feel, what you think and what you do, are properly processed and relayed. They also control things you are barely aware of, the bodily functions which, though on "automatic pilot," keep you alive. These include breathing, heart rate, blood pressure, and bladder and bowel elimination. The spinal cord is the senior VP, the liaison between the nerve passageways in the body and the brain. The brain itself is the CEO, translating information, delegating action, regulating activity, and keeping things organized and easily retrieved.

The motor nerves work the "big picture," your movement, your breathing, your body's regulation. The sensory nerves provide the way we view and react to that big picture. They send messages to the brain, which interprets what we see, feel, hear, taste, and touch.

Spinal cord injury usually occurs without brain injury. The mind remains crystal clear, but it cannot send or receive messages from the nerve passageways through the spinal column, such as instructions to walk, to eliminate the bladder, or to raise your arm. But 35% of spinal cord injuries do involve some degree of brain injury which, overshadowed by the dramatic symptoms of the SCI, can go unnoticed for weeks or even several months. Here, you, the survivor, might start feeling strange; you might find you cannot control your emotions. You, the caregiver, may observe that your loved one is acting overly loud or flamboyant. He might begin to say or do things that are embarrassing. Her depression might worsen.

SPINAL CORDS

SCI MYTH #1:
PEOPLE WITH SCI CANNOT LEAD AN ACTIVE LIFE

Don't mention this one around anyone participating in the Paralympics or to the office colleague who may have the cubicle next to yours. Today, having a spinal cord injury doesn't limit the sports you can enjoy — from skydiving to kayaking, from bicycling to skiing — or the career path you choose. You'll find people with SCI in every profession and industry. They are attorneys, teachers, accountants, plant managers, truck drivers, race car drivers, electrical engineers, and beauty consultants! Yes, there are adjustments to be made, but with rehabilitation and adaptive equipment now available, a person can lead a full, active life without the use of his arms or legs. Simple adjustments at home or in the workplace, including ramps and disabled-accessible parking spaces can usually be completed inexpensively and quickly.

*A final note: Wheelchairs should not be viewed as prisons — by patients or the world at large. When you see a person in a wheelchair, it does not mean she is bound to be in that chair all day long. You might see her next playing with her children on the floor of her den. Sprawled out on the couch reading a book. Floating in the water at the local Y. Or sleeping peacefully under her warm, down comforter. Wheelchairs, as with other equipment, are tools. Like hospital beds, bathtub bars, and motorized lifts, they are designed to help a person with SCI lead as normal a life as possible. They are only a facet of someone's life, **not** life itself.*

A CORD IS A CORD IS A CORD

Like any valuable, priceless treasure, the spinal cord needs protection to keep harm at bay. That's where the skeletal bony frame called the spine, or the backbone, comes in. It is made up of blocks, one on top of another, called vertebrae. Each vertebra is thickest in front; each arches up and away in the back.

To keep your now protected spinal column flexible, there are intervertebral discs between each vertebra. These discs, made of gelatinous material, are the culprits in those ubiquitous "slipped discs" that may cause backache complaints. These intervertebral discs help absorb shock; they act as a cushion for the vertebrae stacked above and below.

The spinal cord, all 18 inches of it, runs through and down these stacked vertebrae and intervertebral discs:

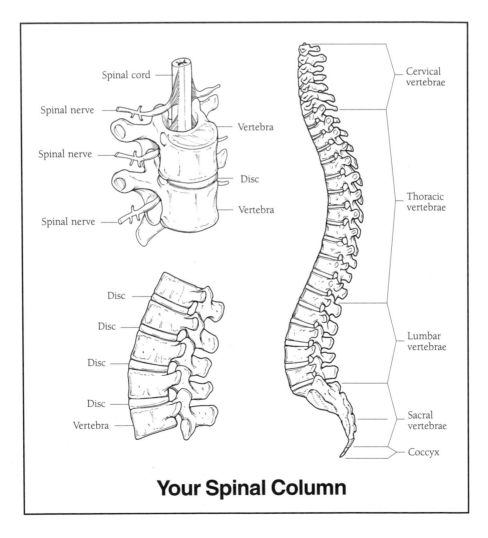

Spinal cord

Spinal nerve

Vertebra

Spinal nerve

Disc

Vertebra

Spinal nerve

Cervical vertebrae

Thoracic vertebrae

Lumbar vertebrae

Disc

Disc

Disc

Disc

Vertebra

Sacral vertebrae

Coccyx

Your Spinal Column

√ The "Top Seven" in vertebrae language are the cervical vertebrae, or C1 to C7, starting with the first one at the base of the skull.

√ The next group, the 12 thoracics, follows from the bottom of the neck, through the chest, to the curve of the back. These "blocks," also numbered from highest to lowest, go from T1 to T12.

√ The lower back contains both the lumbar vertebrae, all five of them, L1 to L5, and the five sacrals, fused together in the "tailbone" (S1 to S5). This image of a tail is truer than you might think. The nerves of the spinal cord continue beyond the bony vertebrae. The spinal cord ends at L2. The remaining nerves, dubbed the cauda equina, "hang down" like a horse's tail from the lumbar and sacral regions.

NERVES OF STEEL

The spinal cord, encased in its cozy vertebrae "home," not only receives and sends messages to and from the outlying nerve passageways, the peripheral nervous system, it is also made up of nerves that travel to and from the brain. These "brain-bound" bundles of spinal nerves stem from the brain to the waist; they move muscles, joints, and limbs with the help of "orders from above": the brain.

There are also spinal nerve fibers that branch out into the peripheral nervous system *between* the vertebrae. They can move muscles, joints, and limbs without "bothering the brain." The spinal column itself can process the sensation they are relaying and send out an appropriate response in less than the time it takes for you to say "back." Examples of this "no-brainer" include all muscular reflex action, such as the "knee-jerk reaction" that occurs when your doctor lightly hits your knee with a medical hammer to test your reflexes during a physical exam.

Here's a sampling of how the nerves of the spinal column work in unison with the brain:

You are in your kitchen, waiting for the water to boil in the teapot. You're impatient. You can't wait for that cup of tea. Finally, at last, the whistle blows. You grab the teapot and begin to pour. In your hurry, you neglect to notice that the top of the teapot isn't securely in place. As you pour, the lid falls off and boiling-hot water drips all over your hand. Ouch! You scream. You shake your hand. The brain receives the sensation from the peripheral nerves: Hot! It sends out a message to react through the spinal column. The spinal cord nerves, in turn, immediately send out a response: Shake and move that hand! All this in an instant. And, within the next few seconds, the brain calls to arms. You forget that song you were singing, that brilliant business ploy, the menu you were planning for dinner. Now all thoughts — and action — are involved in cleaning up the mess, administering first aid to your hand, and discovering new curse words under your breath (not necessarily in this order)!

But suppose the stimulus from the outside world is more complicated than hot or cold, dry or wet. Suppose you are walking down the steps of your back deck with your arms full of garbage bags, and you stumble on the next-to-last step. You begin to fall. You *know* you are going to fall. Your brain is actively involved, sending messages back and forth through your spinal column and out to your body. You're scared. The ground is slippery. The slate slabs below are hard. You can seriously hurt yourself. Immediately, the brain sends the order: Drop the garbage and put out your arms to cushion the fall. The nerves within the spinal column relay the message to your muscles. Your arms move out; garbage falls through the sky. You fall, but your arms protect your head and chest. You'll be black and blue, but nothing more. Here, in less than a millisecond, the entire nervous system, from the brain on down, joined forces to make a brilliant, if not graceful, maneuver.

But what if your spinal column is injured? What if the nerves are damaged at the place of impact and a message cannot be relayed or received from the brain?

FUNCTION EQUALS FORM

When you injure your spinal cord, its bundle of nerves become swollen, bruised, or severed, resulting in a lack of communication between nerve pathways.

When people hear that "your spinal cord is not severed," it gives them false hope, as if it can be repaired. It's important to remember: Most injuries do not result in a severed spinal cord. Your nerves are damaged and your new situation is usually permanent. The brain can no longer detect movement; its orders are ignored by both the muscles and nerves below the injury site. Peripheral nerves can no longer send messages that require immediate action: Too hot! Too cold! Ouch! Like a short circuit or a blown fuse, the spinal column at the place of impact on down remains silent. Nor can the brain order a leg to move away, up, down, or across. The leg receives no messages, no sensations. Nothing.

The severity of this silence depends on the site of spinal cord injury. Physicians can determine exactly what functions will be affected by the extent of nerve damage at a particular level:

- C1 through T1, for example, will result in a quadriplegic injury, involving the neck, arm muscles, chest, abdomen, legs, and diaphragm. Bowel and bladder capabilities will be affected. Both arms and legs will be paralyzed. A person injured here may need help in breathing. He will need some help for

Functional Activities

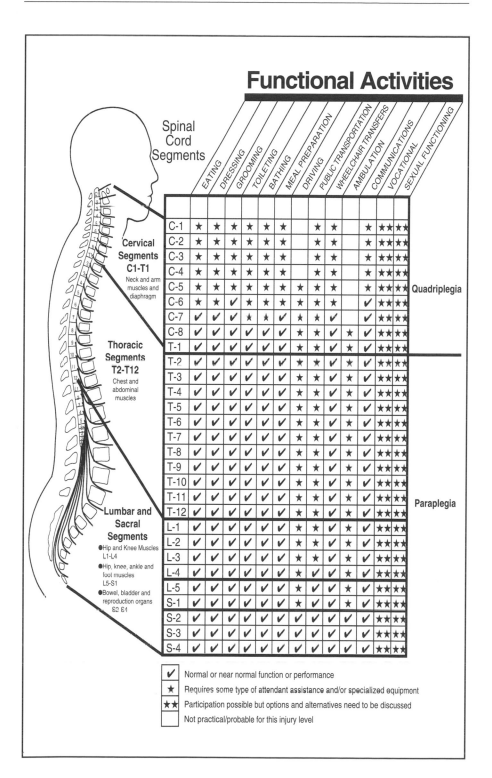

Spinal Cord Segments

Cervical Segments C1-T1 — Neck and arm muscles and diaphragm

Thoracic Segments T2-T12 — Chest and abdominal muscles

Lumbar and Sacral Segments
- Hip and Knee Muscles L1-L4
- Hip, knee, ankle and foot muscles L5-S1
- Bowel, bladder and reproduction organs S2-S4

Spinal Cord Segment	EATING	DRESSING	GROOMING	TOILETING	BATHING	MEAL PREPARATION	DRIVING	PUBLIC TRANSPORTATION	WHEELCHAIR TRANSFERS	AMBULATION	COMMUNICATIONS	VOCATIONAL FUNCTIONING	SEXUAL FUNCTIONING	
C-1	★	★	★	★	★	★		★	★		★	★★	★★	
C-2	★	★	★	★	★	★		★	★		★	★★	★★	
C-3	★	★	★	★	★	★		★	★		★	★★	★★	
C-4	★	★	★	★	★	★		★	★		★	★★	★★	
C-5	★	★	★	★	★	★	★	★	★		★	★★	★★	Quadriplegia
C-6	★	★	✔	★	★	★	★	★	★		✔	★★	★★	
C-7	✔	✔	✔	★	★	✔	★	★	✔		✔	★★	★★	
C-8	✔	✔	✔	✔	✔	✔	★	★	✔	★	✔	★★	★★	
T-1	✔	✔	✔	✔	✔	✔	★	★	✔	★	✔	★★	★★	
T-2	✔	✔	✔	✔	✔	✔	★	★	✔	★	✔	★★	★★	
T-3	✔	✔	✔	✔	✔	✔	★	★	✔	★	✔	★★	★★	
T-4	✔	✔	✔	✔	✔	✔	★	★	✔	★	✔	★★	★★	
T-5	✔	✔	✔	✔	✔	✔	★	★	✔	★	✔	★★	★★	
T-6	✔	✔	✔	✔	✔	✔	★	★	✔	★	✔	★★	★★	
T-7	✔	✔	✔	✔	✔	✔	★	★	✔	★	✔	★★	★★	
T-8	✔	✔	✔	✔	✔	✔	★	★	✔	★	✔	★★	★★	
T-9	✔	✔	✔	✔	✔	✔	★	★	✔	★	✔	★★	★★	
T-10	✔	✔	✔	✔	✔	✔	★	★	✔	★	✔	★★	★★	
T-11	✔	✔	✔	✔	✔	✔	★	★	✔	★	✔	★★	★★	Paraplegia
T-12	✔	✔	✔	✔	✔	✔	★	★	✔	★	✔	★★	★★	
L-1	✔	✔	✔	✔	✔	✔	★	★	✔	★	✔	★★	★★	
L-2	✔	✔	✔	✔	✔	✔	★	★	✔	★	✔	★★	★★	
L-3	✔	✔	✔	✔	✔	✔	★	★	✔	★	✔	★★	★★	
L-4	✔	✔	✔	✔	✔	✔	★	✔	✔	★	✔	★★	★★	
L-5	✔	✔	✔	✔	✔	✔	★	✔	✔	★	✔	★★	★★	
S-1	✔	✔	✔	✔	✔	✔	★	✔	✔	★	✔	★★	★★	
S-2	✔	✔	✔	✔	✔	✔	✔	✔	✔	✔	✔	★★	★★	
S-3	✔	✔	✔	✔	✔	✔	✔	✔	✔	✔	✔	★★	★★	
S-4	✔	✔	✔	✔	✔	✔	✔	✔	✔	✔	✔	★★	★★	

Legend:

✔	Normal or near normal function or performance
★	Requires some type of attendant assistance and/or specialized equipment
★★	Participation possible but options and alternatives need to be discussed
(blank)	Not practical/probable for this injury level

his activities of daily living that use muscles, organs, and nerve passageways below the level of injury. Here, this can mean anything from using a wheelchair to getting dressed, from combing his hair to eating or speaking. However, if the injury is at the C7 - T1 level, a person is usually independent; they are mobile and able to perform their everyday activities.

- T2 through T12 will result in a paraplegic injury. A person will have full use of his arms, but an injury here will affect the legs, the chest, and the abdominal muscles. It may also create bladder and bowel complications. A person with, say, a T10 injury will probably need a wheelchair. He will most likely need adaptive equipment to drive a car.

- L1 through S1 may or may not create paraplegic symptoms. Injuries here involve the hip and lower leg muscles, as well as the bladder and bowel. She may need braces to walk. He may have impotence. People with injuries in this locale are usually taught successfully how to walk again.

- S2 through S4 injuries create a much more focused disability than those that occur "higher up the spinal scale." Damage here does not rule out walking. But it can still create bladder and bowel complications, as well as problems in the bedroom.

(See the chart on page 11 on the spinal cord for an exact description of shape, location, and affected function for all these injury sites.)

Congratulations! You have just learned the basics about the spinal cord and the nuts and bolts of spinal cord injury. But more than knowing about locale is necessary for accurate diagnosis. *How much* damage is as important as *where*. In the next chapter, we'll examine diagnosis and the ways it influenced treatment since primitive times.

DIAGNOSIS AND EARLY TREATMENT

"I knew what I had. I couldn't move my legs. I was paralyzed. But the diagnostic tests my doctor ordered showed me that it was much deeper than that. It isn't always, 'Crash! You'll never walk again.' It turned out my condition was treatable with rehabilitation, and I have learned to walk with a cane. I've also found something really important: hope."

– A 20-year-old student who had an accident
white-water rafting down
the Colorado River

Just for a moment, go back in time. The year is 1700 B.C. Imagine yourself as an Egyptian citizen in a white sheath and colorful headdress, a physician's apprentice taking notes on a piece of just-formed papyrus. A worker is brought into your tent; he was injured carrying stone to the pyramids. He cannot move his legs. He cannot move his arms.

The wise physician orders a treatment including binding the spine and torso with meat, and applying grease to the neck and forehead. Honey should be massaged into his damaged areas daily. But, even as you write these words down, you know what the physician really thinks, what Egyptians had decided almost 5,000 years ago: "Spinal injury cannot be treated."

SLOW GOINGS

Unfortunately, inroads into spinal cord injury treatment have not progressed with much speed throughout much of history. The ancient Greeks and Romans invented a type of treatment dubbed succussion. Here, the injured person was literally tied to an upright pole which was then shaken violently. Whether this methodology was to "shake the nerves to wake up," realign the spinal column, or just something the Greeks could do to try to help, is not sure. But one thing is certain: It didn't help. In fact, it most likely caused more damage.

The spinal cord injured didn't fare any better in the Middle Ages. Physicians actually performed surgery (without any anesthesia stronger than wine) to try to remove the bone fragments they were sure were irritating the nerves and causing problems.

Needless to say, this also didn't help. The Renaissance had the right idea about stress relief and, if muscle tension was the reason for paralysis, they might have hit on something, making the likes of Leonardo da Vinci proud: They applied pressure to the neck and shoulders in a rudimentary traction. Unfortunately, spinal cord injury is not simply a case of a sprained muscle. In most cases, the spinal column encased in the vertebrae is badly damaged. It needs time and life adjustment as treatment, not just traction or a heating pad.

Things got so bad for the spinal-cord injured that by World War I, most soldiers who suffered from some form of spinal cord injury died within weeks, usually through complications arising from their condition: urinary infections, pneumonia and respiratory ailments, pressure sores, and soaring high blood pressure. Even with the advent of neurosurgery, the prospects for spinal cord injury victims looked dismal unless survivors only had mild damage to their nerves.

REHABILITATION JUMP-START

By World War II, the situation had become increasingly serious. More and more soldiers were coming into the makeshift hospitals, the air bombs zooming overhead, complaining of spinal injuries. They couldn't walk. They couldn't breathe. They couldn't move their arms. Indeed, there were more cases of SCI than death on arrival to the camps.

Clearly, something had to be done. Enter one Sir Ludwig Guttmann, the physician considered the father of modern rehabilitation. Before he began his work at the Stoke Mandeville Hospital in England, the spinal-cord injured were considered victims in the worst sense. They were placed in hospitals, alone and desolate, while physicians and nurses waited for them to die. There was a stigma attached to these people; prejudice abounded, even among the staff.

But Sir Ludwig believed that these people, with their active minds intact, could be retrieved from a terrible self-defeating fate. He believed that if they were introduced to a way of adapting to their new life, they could find renewed purpose in living. They could find hope and become active, thriving members of society. To accomplish this goal, he set up rehabilitation teams and voiced the necessity for long-range care if these people should become well.

It was Sir Ludwig who made people understand that bladder and bowel problems, pressure sores, and infection were natural results of the immobility of spinal cord injury. He introduced catheterization and, along with his top-notch team of physicians, therapists, counselors, and even school teachers, helped to dispel the myths that had kept the spinal-cord injured feeling like victims.

At the same time, medical and scientific advances were being made in treating and diagnosing spinal cord injury. Medications were introduced that could halt the advancement of injury if given during the first few hours of the accident. Antibiotics kept infections at bay; antidepressants helped ease the depression that inevitably came with the realization of the full extent of injury.

Wheelchairs, too, were making new inroads into mobility. With special electrical switches, equipment, and even chairs designed for almost any sport, there was no reason why spinal cord injury survivors could not become — and remain — flourishing, contributing members of society.

VITAL CLUES

But before successful rehabilitation can begin, the injury itself must be diagnosed. The rehabilitation team must determine the extent of the damage — and exactly where on the spinal column the injury took place. They must determine the injured person's ability to function in daily life; they must determine how much sensation they have, what they can feel, and where. And, during the rehabilitation treatment, progress must continually be monitored — in order to change, to correct, to advance — for the best possible rehabilitation.

SPINAL CORDS

REGENERATION FOR THE NEXT GENERATION?

It's an old axiom: Central nervous system nerves cannot regenerate. Once you have a spinal cord injury, you have it for life. But change is afoot. Nerves in the outlying peripheral nervous system do grow back, so why not the spinal cord? Scientists are now discovering that perhaps, someday, it will be possible to see growth. Instead of concentrating on the fibers themselves, they are experimenting with the environment. When laboratory animals were given the proper foundation (additional cells that act like "glue magnets" for the damaged nerve fibers) and growth factors, they did experience the return of some function.

It's too soon to tell if this will prove to be the case for humans, but the initial studies sound promising.

The first step in diagnosis is determining the exact type of spinal cord injury that has occurred:

Injurious Acts #1: Flexion Injury

Spinal cord injury does not occur in a vacuum. When something happens to the nerves in the spinal column, chances are there are injuries to either the surrounding bony vertebrae, the discs, or the ligaments and muscles around the spinal column. A flexion injury means that a person, say, fell off a horse and their spinal column is literally thrust forward or sideways. Not only is there nerve damage, but part of the vertebrae can be broken and pushed out of alignment; surrounding ligaments can be ripped. The spinal column is no longer straight, the vertebrae lined up one on top of the other; it is distorted.

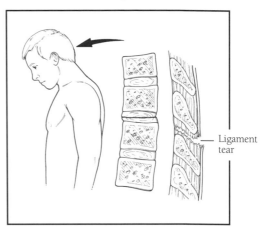

Injurious Acts #2: Hyperextension Injury

You're driving in your car. Suddenly, a truck appears in front of you and you hit the brakes just in time to avoid a head-on collision. But, crash! The car behind you, moving just as fast, slams into your rear bumper. Hard. Fast. On impact, your body is actually bent backward, including your spinal column. This "hit from the rear" incident is a hyperextension type of spinal injury and may involve torn discs and ligaments, including the compressed, distorted, badly misaligned nerves of the spinal column.

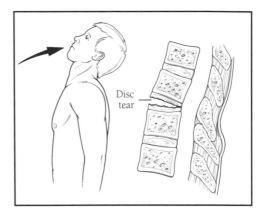

Injurious Acts #3: Compression Injury

A worst case scenario: You're on a construction site, up on the frame of a third-story home. You lose your balance on the railing and fall on your buttocks — right on a ladder that's set up below. Whoosh! The fall hits you hard, "squeezing" your spinal column together, shortening your vertebrae. In other words, the force of the fall created a compression injury, which presses down on your spinal cord, not only hurting the nerves, but smashing the covering vertebrae.

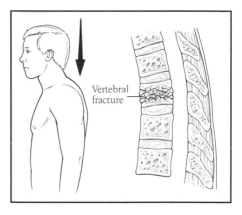

Injurious Acts #4: Rotation Injury

You've bundled the kids into the van. The dog, as usual, is in the back, looking out the rear window. But traffic is heavy; your nerves are frazzled; and the kids are screaming at each other — all over the din of the barking dog. Without thinking, you quickly turn your head as you get into the right lane. You start to shout

for quiet just as a Jeep crashes into the side of your van. Boom! The van jangles, vibrates. You are hit hard from the driver's side. In this type of "sideswipe" spinal cord injury, you've suddenly twisted your spinal cord in different directions at the same time. Vertebrae can snap; nerves can be stretched and severed.

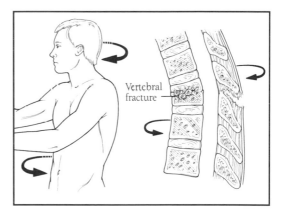

SPINAL CORDS

THE SHOCKING TRUTH

When you first have a spinal cord injury, the trauma to your system can make your condition seem worse than it really is. You might experience paralysis, a loss of reflexes, numbness, a drop in blood pressure, loss of bladder and bowel control, even irregular breathing — but it might not be permanent. It might be a condition called spinal shock which can stay around for days or weeks. Once your body adjusts, you might regain some muscle activity and some sensory control. As your spinal shock evolves, your hospital team can perform a much more accurate assessment of your condition.

Injurious Acts #5: An Incomplete Injury

Incomplete is exactly how it sounds: partial, not total. Whether your accident results in a compression, rotation, hyperextension, or flexion injury, if you are able to move any muscle or feel something, anything, below the level where you were injured, you have an incomplete SCI.

A *central cord incomplete injury* means that the center of the spinal cord has been damaged and, depending on the exact locale, may selectively involve the arms more than the legs.

Central Cord Syndrome

If your accident involved an *upper section of the spinal cord* that moves the arms, you may lose movement in both your upper and your lower body.

If it involved a *lower section of the spinal cord,* you may have more difficulty walking. You may also have problems with your bladder and bowels.

Anterior Spinal Cord Syndrome

An *anterior spinal cord incomplete injury* means the accident involved the front section of the spinal cord. You will lose all movement below the level of injury, but you may be able to feel: touch, vibrations, hot, or cold.

A *posterior spinal cord incomplete injury* is just the opposite of the anterior; it involves the back section of the spinal nerves. You may be able to move, regardless of the point of injury, although you may lose the sense of movement. You will move but you might not be able to feel it.

Posterior Spinal Cord Syndrome

A *Brown-Sequard incomplete injury* involves one-half of the spinal cord. You won't feel or be able to move below the level of injury, but

Brown-Sequard Syndrome

only on the side where the injury occurred. However, sensation, such as hot, cold, and pain, will be gone on the *opposite side* where the injury occurred.

Injurious Acts #6: Complete Injury

Complete is just that, complete. However the injury occurred, whatever the type, if your SCI is complete, it is total. (You don't need to have a severed spinal cord to have a complete injury.) Spinal nerves are completely damaged. You will not feel anything or be able to move below the level of injury.

SPINAL CORDS

A WINDOW OF OPPORTUNITY

The first 12 hours after a spinal cord injury are the most crucial. If powerful steroids are given in the acute-care hospital, swelling, inflammation, and bruising will be reduced, preventing the injury from getting worse. Studies performed by the National Institutes of Health found that the drug methylprednisolone helped reduce the severity of paralysis if given during this "window of opportunity." The only exception? Completely severed spinal cord nerves, which rarely occurs.

TEST MOVES

It's easy to look at a drawing and point to the type of injury it illuminates. But it's quite another when it's your body — or someone's you love — at stake. Knowing the type of injury, the severity, its repercussions, is vital, not only for correct acute trauma care, but for rehabilitation to progress and be successful.

Fortunately, we've come a long way from the days of makeshift traction and the pole shaking of succussion. Diagnosis is no longer a magician's trick. Although not quite as fast as pulling a rabbit out of a hat, today's diagnostic tools are more accurate — and faster — than ever before. Here's a sampling:

- **X-ray:** Yes, that simple test you had when your arm broke, when you sprained your ankle, when you went for your last checkup. Safer and more accurate than ever, thanks to better-quality film and technology, an X-ray still offers a clear, concise picture of your bones, specifically your vertebrae, that can help a physician determine whether your accident caused a fracture or dislocation.

- **CT Scan:** You can call this CAT (**C**omputerized **A**xial **T**omography), but never call it a "dog." The CT scan goes where X-rays only dared to go and is now a familiar sight in many hospitals and clinics. This large, doughnut-shaped machine takes pictures of the spinal column, photographically "slicing" open the body to reveal the damage to the bones in a much more detailed, precise manner.

- **MRI:** No, this is not a new form of salutation. The initials actually stand for Magnetic Resonance Imaging and, like its kin, the CT scan, is now a familiar diagnostic device in hospitals and clinics. MRI takes accuracy one step further. A combination of computer technology and physics, MRIs use radio frequencies and a magnet to chart electrical charges as they surge

---

SPINAL CORDS

"The Doors of Wisdom are never shut."
– Benjamin Franklin

There is always something to learn if you — or a loved one — have a spinal cord injury.

---

through the spinal cord. It then converts these charges into computerized, highly detailed pictures which clearly and efficiently display damage done to the spinal cord. While a CT scan is better for bones, an MRI is the test of choice for the discs and soft tissue or the spinal cord itself, which is so small that a CT scan simply won't show it as well.

- *Neurological and Neuropsychological Testing:* These tests literally get to the heart of the matter. Both muscles (from your quadriceps to your triceps, from your biceps to your finger abductors) and sensory points (using a slight prick from a safety pin at various spots on your body, including your fingers, heel, thigh, and toes) are evaluated and given a grade. This helps determine severity of injury as well as the right rehabilitation. *(See the next section, "ASIA MAJOR," for a more thorough look at this important diagnostic tool.)*

Neuropsychological tests help determine if you have any brain injury (Remember: 35% of all SCI also involve the head) via questions that test your memory, your ability to differentiate right from left, your ability to speak and understand language, your perceptions of the world around you, and your behavior. These tests also help determine the level of depression you might be suffering.

- *The Ashworth Scale:* It's one thing to clench your hands in anticipation or flex your toes to ease tired feet — and quite another when those muscles clench and tighten by themselves. Spasticity, or abnormally increased muscle tone, is a common side effect of paralysis. *(The opposite of spasticity is atrophy, or flaccid muscles, another side effect that is covered in chapter four.)* It can be a very real problem in spinal cord injury, not only hindering physical therapy and interfering with the activities of daily living, but also causing pain. To describe and document the amount of spasticity that is involved, health professionals use the Ashworth Scale. Each muscle's tone is tested, including range of motion, muscle strength, flexing, and releasing. The Ashworth Scale is used throughout rehabilitation as an evaluation tool.

SPINAL CORDS

THE ASIA DEGREE OF IMPAIRMENT SCALE

A: Complete Injury. *You have no feeling or motor function below the level of injury, including the sacral segments of the spinal cord, the genitals, and the rectal area.*

B: Incomplete Injury. *(Preserved sensation only) Your ability to feel is not completely lost, but you have no motor function below the level of injury. (This also includes the genital and rectal areas.)*

C: Incomplete Injury. *(Some sensory and motor function preserved) You have some muscle control (although not normal) below the level of injury. When key muscles in this area are tested, more than half register lower than a muscle grade of 3.*

D: Incomplete Injury. *(Preserved motor function) You have fair muscle control below the level of injury. When key muscles in this area are tested, more than half are greater or equal to a muscle grade of 3.*

E: Normal. *Both your sensory and motor functions are completely normal.*

- **FIM:** No, this is not a typo in a Discovery Channel listing about the sea. FIM stands for Functional Independence Measures and, more than any other diagnostic tool, it details the impact the spinal cord injury has on your life. In other words, this test helps determine your ability to carry out the functions of daily living: dressing, grooming, bathing, eating, communicating, and getting around town. Developed at the State University of New York (SUNY) in Buffalo, it involves 18 areas (including those above) which are constantly upgraded and evaluated during rehabilitation. Each of the 18 activities is given its own classification: from 7 (total independence) through 5 (supervised self-care, such as using adaptive equipment to dress) to 1 (total assistance to perform the activity).

ASIA MAJOR

Clarity is vital in any field, in any relationship, in any situation, but when it comes to health, clear communication is a matter of life and death. Spinal cord injury is no exception. Clarity is vital for proper diagnosis, as well as determining the right — and most successful — rehabilitation. Standards must be set that can be communicated to an entire rehabilitation team, that can be used to describe an injury fast and in terms that everyone involved can understand. This standard now exists. Designed by the American Spinal

---

SPINAL CORDS

MOTOR GRADING SCALE

0 = *Total paralysis*
1 = *Visible or palpable contraction*
2 = *Active movement with full range of motion. No movement against gravity.*
3 = *Active movement with full range of motion. Against gravity.*
4 = *Active movement with full range of motion. Moderate resistance added.*
5 = *Normal. Active movement with full range of motion. Full resistance added.*
NT = *Not testable.*

Injury Association (ASIA), it is a chart of neurological classification, pinpointing both sensation and the ability to move. Called the ASIA classification, it is not only useful in describing an injury in clear, universal language, but it is also a help in establishing and tracking progress during acute care and rehabilitation.

Here's an example:

Jonathan was rushed to the ER, unable to move his right leg. An X-ray and a CT scan showed that he had a fracture of his L1 vertebra (the bone that encases the spinal cord). Neurological testing showed that he could move his right leg slightly, but that he could not feel it. He could not move his left side at all. He also lost control of his bladder and bowels. Jonathan's injury was given the identification R-L1M (for right lumbar 1 motor ability).

As it happened, Jonathan's skeletal and neurological injury were at the same level, but this can vary. The fracture may be at C4 level, but the neurological damage may not start until C6. In other words, you can have a fracture at a different level than your neurological damage. Your neck can break, but the neurological damage may not happen for an inch further down your spinal column. Further, depending on the injury site, your left or right side may be stronger — or weaker. In Jonathan's case, his left side proved to be worse than his right; he couldn't move his left arm or leg, but he had limited ability on his right side.

If you have difficulty understanding this concept, think of the last time you gripped a garden hose. The water might have continued to flow an inch or two higher up than where your hand held the hose. You also might have noticed that the water flowed faster from the left side of the spout than the right, or vice versa, depending on your hand's grip.

STANDARD NEUROLOGICAL CLASSIFICATION OF SPINAL CORD INJURY

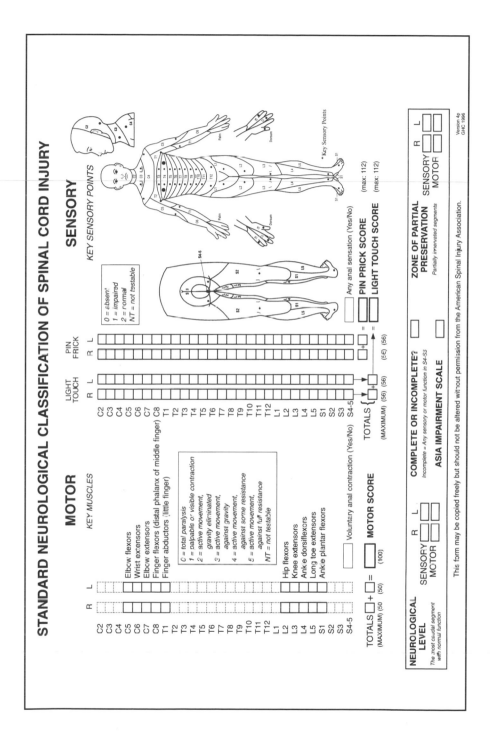

MOTOR

KEY MUSCLES

R	L	
		C2
		C3
		C4
		C5 Elbow flexors
		C6 Wrist extensors
		C7 Elbow extensors
		C8 Finger flexors (distal phalanx of middle finger)
		T1 Finger abductors (little finger)
		T2
		T3
		T4
		T5
		T6
		T7
		T8
		T9
		T10
		T11
		T12
		L1
		L2 Hip flexors
		L3 Knee extensors
		L4 Ankle dorsiflexors
		L5 Long toe extensors
		S1 Ankle plantar flexors
		S2
		S3
		S4-5

0 = total paralysis
1 = palpable or visible contraction
2 = active movement,
     gravity eliminated
3 = active movement,
     against gravity
4 = active movement,
     against some resistance
5 = active movement,
     against full resistance
NT = not testable

Voluntary anal contraction (Yes/No) ☐

☐ **MOTOR SCORE**

TOTALS ☐ + ☐ = ☐ (100)
(MAXIMUM) (50) (50)

SENSORY

KEY SENSORY POINTS

LIGHT TOUCH		PIN PRICK	
R	L	R	L
	C2		
	C3		
	C4		
	C5		
	C6		
	C7		
	C8		
	T1		
	T2		
	T3		
	T4		
	T5		
	T6		
	T7		
	T8		
	T9		
	T10		
	T11		
	T12		
	L1		
	L2		
	L3		
	L4		
	L5		
	S1		
	S2		
	S3		
	S4-5		

0 = absent†
1 = impaired
2 = normal
NT = not testable

Any anal sensation (Yes/No) ☐

TOTALS { ☐ + ☐ (56) } = ☐ **PIN PRICK SCORE** (max: 112)
(MAXIMUM) (56) (56)
{ ☐ + ☐ (56) } = ☐ **LIGHT TOUCH SCORE** (max: 112)

* Key Sensory Points

NEUROLOGICAL LEVEL		COMPLETE OR INCOMPLETE?		ZONE OF PARTIAL PRESERVATION	
The most caudal segment with normal function	SENSORY ☐ R ☐ L	Incomplete = Any sensory or motor function in S4-S5		Partially innervated segments	SENSORY ☐ R ☐ L
	MOTOR ☐ R ☐ L	**ASIA IMPAIRMENT SCALE** ☐			MOTOR ☐ R ☐ L

This form may be copied freely but should not be altered without permission from the American Spinal Injury Association.

Version 4p
GHC 1996

23

The reason for this differentiation? *The ASIA system uses the neurological level for rating the injury.*

ASIA goes even deeper in determining a person's spinal cord injury. Muscle tone, too, is classified on a scale of 0 through 5. *(See the chart, "Motor Grading Scale," on page 22.)* As Jonathan could move his right leg against gravity (without sensory information going up to the brain), he was given a grade of 3: fair.

Jonathan's injury was classified as incomplete, with some motor function intact, and sensory ability lost below the L1 point of injury. His rehabilitation would include bladder and bowel management, as well as learning to walk again with braces.

Congratulations! You've finished your "test" and you are ready to begin your rehabilitation, taking that first step towards your new, independent life — and a new understanding of hope, help, and realistic goals.

CHAPTER THREE

A REHABILITATION EDUCATION: AN OVERVIEW

- *What's the use of rehabilitation? I can't move my legs. I won't ever be able to move my legs. So forget it! WRONG!*

- *A spinal cord injury is hopeless. Better to just resign yourself to a lifetime of dependency and depression. WRONG!*

- *Rehabilitation hospitals are cold, uncaring places. I'd rather be at home, not being able to leave my bed, than be just another number in an institution. WRONG!*

- *Rehabilitation is rehabilitation. It doesn't matter where you go or what the staff is like. They're all the same: a doctor, some nurses, and a therapist. WRONG!*

- *I don't want rehabilitation. I want to walk just the way I did before. Nothing less will do. I want to walk now! WRONG!*

If you or someone you love has recently suffered a spinal cord injury, you probably have heard misguided comments like these — and others very similar. Let's face it: Rehabilitation is not something you seek information about unless you have to. It's not something we like to dwell on.

The idea of rehabilitation is also fraught with anxiety, confusion, and trauma. More times than not, you are not in an ideal state of mind to make an informed decision. You are hopeful, but, at the same time, there are all those myths.

RESTORE, NOT CURE

Rehabilitation is not a cure. It's not take these two pills and call me in the morning. It's not get a lot of bed rest and within a few months, you'll be as good as new. Rehabilitation is all about helping you help yourself to make profound changes, to explore new avenues of thinking, believing, and doing things to achieve the independence that is within your reach. Rather than a cure, it is a process designed to restore your life. A good rehabilitation hospital will help you or your loved one achieve as much independence as possible.

GETTING PEOPLE BACK: THE FACTS DON'T LIE

Whatever myths you've heard, the fact is that the *right* rehabilitation works. It has a profound influence on injury. When a hospital uses a team approach, where therapists all work together, where the whole is greater than its parts, hospital stays for people with spinal cord injuries have decreased from an average of 134 days to anywhere from 99 to 54 days, depending on the extent of injury. Even better, these stays cost substantially less than in 1973. More good news: Many of these survivors have gone on to lead productive and fairly independent lives. Only 3.1% SCI survivors in one study ended up in nursing homes when their rehabilitation stay was over. And that number dropped to 2% after one year.

TEAMWORK: A MODEL SYSTEM
FOR REHABILITATION — AND LIFE

Independence. *Your* independence. That is the goal of each and every member of the rehabilitation team, from the physical therapist to the vocational therapist, from the dietitian to the case manager.

Not only do team players have their own roles, their own areas of expertise to help enhance a specific aspect of injury, but all of them work together so that progress can remain constant in all areas. A physical therapist will help you learn how to use a particular type of wheelchair while conferring with your physiatrist, neurosurgeon, and rehabilitation nurse on your bladder and bowel progress. A vocational therapist will help you prepare for a new career while conferring with your psychologist on your emotional adaptability.

In other words, each therapist works with you individually, to keep you focused and help you learn as much as possible from their skills.

But, at the same time, they are working with other members of the team to ensure continued overall progress. This total integration of talent and skills makes for the best rehabilitation — which translates into the best treatment for you.

Let's go over these "team players" now:

A Real-Life "Starship Commander": The Rehabilitation Physician

Think of central booking. The captain of the helm. The chief of staff. This is the physiatrist, neurologist, orthopaedic surgeon, or neurosurgeon — all specially trained in the care of the spinal cord. He is responsible for the medical care an SCI patient gets during rehabilitation. She creates the individual

---

SPINAL CORDS

THE REHABILITATION CREDO

In knowledge, there is strength...to accept.
And with that acceptance:
- *You are better motivated to succeed*
- *Your rehabilitation progress stays constant*
- *Your caregivers, if needed, are better able to cope with their new responsibilities — and help you more.*

---

rehabilitation program designed especially for you, following up with the other members of the team and ordering specific therapies and medicines.

A One and a Two and a Three: The Physical Therapist

The PT, as she is called at the rehabilitation hospital, is one of the most important members of the team. It is the PT who most closely teaches independence by helping the SCI survivor regain and maximize available strength in muscles and joints. And, if you need to be on a ventilator, the PT, in tandem with the occupational therapist (*see below*) will help you adapt to new environmental control units (ECU), such as equipment to turn lights on and off, watch television, and go from one room in your house to another. The PT will also show you how to:
- Use your wheelchair
- Safely transfer from bed to chair, from floor to chair, from chair to car
- Handle a specially equipped car or van
- Regain or increase muscle strength
- Turn over and be able to sit up, roll, and be mobile in bed
- Stand, when possible, and walk, if possible

The City Never Sleeps: The Rehabilitation Nurse

Twenty-four-hour care. It's one of the crucial elements that makes up a good rehabilitation hospital. And the person who provides this all-important care, whose watchful eye and skill helps keep pressure sores at bay, manage bowel and bladder function, and provides face to face individual education, is the rehabilitation nurse. She observes your progress and passes information along to the other members of the team — whether you are feeling over whelmed or proceeding nicely, whether you are discouraged or ready to take on the world. He helps you do your "homework" from therapy sessions so you achieve your goals faster and more successfully.

Learning by Doing: The Occupational Therapist (OT)

Occupational therapy goes far beyond pottery making and watercolors. An OT is a critical component for independence. She is the one who teaches an SCI survivor how to live independently again. She teaches ways to adapt to what rehabilitation specialists call activities of daily living (ADL). From dressing to combing your hair, bathing to driving a car, bladder and bowel management to eating your meals, you will learn new methods to remain as independent as possible while performing these tasks.

The OT will help you maximize your physical, psychological, and social abilities for you to live a full life. He will also work with the PT to create exercise programs that are best suited for you. She will design splints that, when attached to your arms, will give you increased function. He will work with your family to create a physically accessible environment at home.

Do You Want to Talk About It?: The Speech and Language Pathologist (SP)

If your spinal cord accident occurred near your brainstem, your paralysis might cause swallowing problems. You might have trouble communicating what you want; your speech might be slurred. You might have some brain injury, which may create perception and language problems. The SP works on all your communication difficulties, teaching you methods for getting your desires and needs to others. She will help you adapt to communication computers, if necessary.

Breathe In, Breathe Out: The Respiratory Therapist (RT)

If your SCI occurred in the upper part of your neck, affecting your breathing, a respiratory therapist, or RT, will be called in to teach you how to breathe with a ventilator. The RT is critical to your survival during the early stages of injury. She will help strengthen respiratory muscles. He will help determine the extent of your respiratory damage.

The Ultimate Organizer: The Case Manager

Think of those cartoons where a worker, sitting behind her desk, is busily signing papers, talking on the phone, filing, discussing a situation with people in her office, six arms, 10 hands, all working at once. This is your case manager, managing her job with only two arms and two hands. The case manager helps your family with the complexities of health insurance. He will act as a liaison between the hospital staff and your family, providing hope, education, and understanding to your often overwhelmed loved one. She will also work with your entire rehabilitation team, making sure everyone is in sync, working toward the same goals and making the same progress.

The case manager can be you and your family's most important team player. *Use* her. Listen to her. And ask as many questions as you want. She is there to help.

You Are What You Eat: The Clinical Dietitian

In today's world, a dietitian can be a luxury. Many people seek out dietitians to help them lose weight, to reduce the symptoms of chronic illnesses, or to remain young and strong. But a clinical dietitian is crucial for spinal cord injury survivors. When you injure your spinal cord, your weight can change drastically; you might gain weight or lose too much. In fact, most survivors initially lose up to 20 pounds!

Your skin may lose its tone and break down. The dietitian will assess your unique situation and plan your meals accordingly. She also knows that a specific diet is necessary for proper bowel and bladder management, and she will make sure you eat foods that will keep you regular. He will also keep careful watch over what you eat to make sure there are no food-drug interactions.

A healthy, low-fat diet, rich in fiber from grains, fruits, and vegetables, is particularly important to those with paralysis. Fiber can help:
- Keep your bowels regular
- Help control high blood pressure, a risk for many SCI survivors
- Maintain healthy skin tone and prevent pressure sores

Your dietitian will also help plan eating habits you can keep for life — in the hospital and when you are at home, living more independently.

Food for the Soul: The Psychologist

Your new life situation can be devastating at first. Accepting your new way of life, understanding the possibilities and opportunities that are still out there, waiting, understanding that your limitations do not have to hold you back — all these are areas where your psychologist can help. He can help you through the mourning process as you grieve for your old self. She can help you cope with your new relationships with your family, your friends, your spouse — as well as help them cope with the changes in you. He will work with *all* of you to help ensure your progress and provide necessary stress reduction and relief for everyone. In short, your psychologist is your adjuster, helping you adjust to your disability and your new fact of life. She is a positive force: With hope, motivation, and determination, your entire rehabilitation will be more successful.

Just Do It!: The Vocational Specialist

There is more to life than learning new ways to perform your routines, your daily activities. After you become more familiar with your wheelchair, your braces, your ventilator, you may need to be introduced to a new vocation, a new career, where you can put your skills and talent to use. The vocational specialist will help you find the right job for you. If necessary, he will help you find a new career, one that is more ability-challenged accessible. (Christopher Reeve, for example, went from a star in front of the camera, to an award-winning director *behind* the camera.) He will help reacclimate you to society, instructing you on the ins and outs of disability laws. If you are a student, your vocational specialist will help you with your studies so you don't fall behind while in the rehabilitation hospital.

We're All in This Together: The Rehabilitation Counselor
All aspects of rehabilitation need family support and education for real success, and the rehabilitation counselor helps ensure that the family stays involved. He is there to help assess your social behavior:
- Do you have a history of depression?
- Have you had trouble making friends?
- What education level do you have?
- Had you been a competitive athlete prior to your injury?
- What is your relationship with your family?

The rehabilitation counselor will analyze your answers as well as interview your family to get their feedback. Based on his findings, he will help both you and your family develop realistic goals — both during your stay in the rehabilitation hospital and long term, at home. He will help keep realistic hope alive.

All Work and No Play Makes Jack a Dull Boy: The Recreational Therapist (TR)
There's nothing like a good laugh to keep spirits up and motivation high. There's nothing like fun to prove that life is indeed rich and worth living! But

---

SPINAL CORDS

FIVE GOLDEN REHABILITATION RULES FOR PATIENT CARE

1. *Rehabilitation is a long process.*
2. *Treatment should not focus completely on physical deficits.*
3. *Recreational and vocational therapies are essential.*
4. *Rehabilitation must include and involve the family.*
5. *Therapists must do their work in the steadfast belief that some improvement will occur. There is a wide range of possibilities between immobilization and walking, including strength building, bladder and bowel management, and regaining self-esteem.*

---

tell that to an SCI survivor. If he has been in PT and OT all day, learning how to use a wheelchair on gravel, how to manage his bladder, how to handle combing his hair, it's going to be difficult to find that kernel of hope, that joy, that can make rehabilitation a success. That's where the recreational therapist comes in. She is not a "cockeyed optimist," ready to fill you with easy plati-tudes that don't mean anything. Rather, she is a trained professional ready to realistically help you enjoy what you liked doing before the accident. Yes, *before* the accident.

Where there is a will, there is a way, and she is ready to show you the tools you need to adapt new ways to do the things you love to do. She will help you enjoy recreational activities, such as reading a good book or preparing a meal for company, as well as perform competitive sports — from bowling to biking. He will show you how to get around the town in a wheelchair, from going to the mall to getting to a movie, from going out to dinner to shopping at the supermarket. He will also help you adjust to your neighborhood and your community when you return back home with suggestions and facts about disabled-accessible buildings, support groups, as well as how to become an active participant in your community's disability laws.

These are the basic rehabilitation hospital's "team players." Each one works independently — and together — to give you the best care possible.

- The PT might be teaching you how to use a wheelchair...
- ...At the same time the OT is teaching you how to perform activities of daily living from that wheelchair...
- ...While the TR works on going to a restaurant in that wheelchair...
- ...And, all the while, the rehabilitation counselor is helping you and your family work on accepting that wheelchair as a part of your new life.

The hospitals you investigate might have some variations on these roles, but a good rehabilitation hospital must have this team approach — with these players — to be a success.

But there are other elements that come into "play" when choosing the right rehabilitation hospital....

FAMILY MATTERS

Quality care while in the rehabilitation hospital is critical, but so is the care you get at home and the support you get from your family while you are pro-gressing.

The fact is that spinal cord injury doesn't just happen to you, it happens to your entire family, to those you love and to those you associate with, on the job and among your friends. True, your wife, for example, doesn't need a wheelchair, but she, too, can feel the devastating loss that you are experiencing. This devastation is complicated by guilt, however illogical, that she is fine, walking around, doing errands, while you, the husband she loves, is using a wheelchair.

Your wife can also feel anger at the situation. Worse, she can feel angry at *you* for having had your accident, creating more guilt and even more anger. The resentment builds, especially when everyone seems to be giving you sympathy and ignoring her. A vicious cycle — and one that has broken up more than one marriage.

In short, families need help too. They not only need to be educated in the correct ways to effectively assist you as needed, but they need an education in coping — with the situation, with any problems that come up, and with the tremendous stress that they, too, are experiencing.

With education and support, families can give the love and kindness so necessary for recovery. By taking care of themselves, they are better able to help you. They can provide a healing touch, strong motivation, and even instill real hope — so important on days when you feel as if you want to wheel your chair as far and as fast as you can. (*See chapter eleven, "Helping Your Loved One Means Helping Yourself: Caregiver Relief," for more details on this vital subject.*)

SPINAL CORDS

"Basic rehabilitation is a drag. It teaches you what you learned in the first four years of life — mobility, personal hygiene, avoidance of hazards, muscle development, and other pretty unoriginal stuff. The best thing going for it is that not doing it is much worse than doing it.

"But that's just Rehab 101. If you're in a good place, you can attend a sexuality seminar, learn to drive a car, join group sessions on relationships, self-image, self-presentation, or whatever else needs discussion, receive vocational counseling and training, learn about money sources, get in some recreation and maybe get out on the town and mix with some normies. (They're pretty weird, but you get used to them.) Lots of good information here, and even some good fun. Enter rehabilitation with a full heart.

"Remember that the genuine aim of rehabilitation is to achieve your goals. Tell them what you want to accomplish, show them that you're willing to work, and they'll literally give you the world."

— Barry Corbet, author
Options: Spinal Cord Injury and the Future
Denver: Hirschfeld Press, 1980.

YOUR HOME AWAY FROM HOME

The difference between a good rehabilitation hospital and a poor one? Everything. A good rehabilitation hospital will provide the knowledge and skill, the equipment, the consideration, and the kindness you would expect in your own home. It will be spotlessly clean, well-organized, and have a full, courteous staff readily accessible to answer your questions.

Remember: One visit is worth a thousand brochures, a hundred photographs, tens of hundreds of phone calls. Use your eyes. Trust your instincts. Seeing is truly believing. Think of buying a house. You'd never decide on purchasing a new home without a thorough inspection. Why should a rehabilitation hospital be any different?

And, in the same way you'd examine a house, asking questions of the present owners, the neighbors, the school and community councils, you'd ask questions of the medical director and the staff of any rehabilitation hospital you are interested in. Here are some we've found particularly important, questions which can make or break a successful rehabilitation:

- *Does this facility have a spinal cord injury program?*
  A rehabilitation hospital that handles SCI on a continuous basis will be knowledgeable, up-to-the-minute, and maintain a high standard of quality. It will be able to handle any SCI situations that come up.

- *Does the program have a spinal cord injury education series?*
  A critical part of your success is dependent upon your ability to understand and cope with your new challenges. The facility should provide a formal program to deal with these issues.

- *Does this facility use a "team approach" as their model system of rehabilitation?*
  As we have seen in earlier sections of this chapter, an integrated team approach has proven to be the most successful in rehabilitation efforts. Each member working separately and with the other "players" means that you will be getting consistent, quality care.

- Is *there a spinal cord medical specialist on staff?*
  This doctor may be a physiatrist, neurologist, or any of the other "real-life" Starship commanders mentioned earlier (*see page 26*). What's important here is that the doctor at the helm is trained to coordinate all the rehabilitation programs in his hospital. She is trained to assess damage and determine the best rehabilitation for you. Another crucial point: A good hospital with its "team approach" would definitely have a spinal cord specialist on staff, if not as its "commander."

- *Does the rehabilitation program establish both short-term and long-term goals?*
  A good hospital not only sets realistic "in-house" goals, such as transferring from your bed to your wheelchair within, say, six weeks, walking from your room to the cafeteria with your new braces within, perhaps,

---

SPINAL CORDS

Guilt can bind you and make you helpless. Nowhere is this more true than in spinal cord injury. Many wives and husbands want to take care of their loved one by themselves. They refuse help — and they certainly won't pay anyone to come in and bathe their spouse or help with grooming!

But this spousal guilt can hurt much more than pride. It adds tremendous stress to an already stressful situation. Caregivers can become physically sick and unable to help, or so angry and resentful, they become full-fledged martyrs who no one wants to be around.

The moral? Don't feed bad about hiring a caregiver. Interview and hire without guilt. Accept help gladly. Be the spouse, a husband or wife, not the caregiver. Your loved one will actually thank you for it.

---

three months, but it also sees the future, when you are at home, and sets goals accordingly: learning a new job skill, if necessary; maintaining a relationship; and handling activities of daily living as independently as possible.

• *Does this facility involve the family?*

How much does the family count in this hospital? Do you see the able-bodied walking around the hall, engaging in conversation with staff, acting very comfortable and very much at home? Is there a family-oriented rehabilitation counselor and case manager on staff, one who will be specifically assigned to you? If so, chances are this hospital believes that rehabilitation support means family support. They know that the family can encourage success — or hinder it. They know that the family is as important an element for progress as learning to use a wheelchair. We all need support and understanding from those around us. SCI survivors certainly are no exception.

THE SIX MAIN ARENAS OF
SPINAL CORD INJURY REHABILITATION

You've been introduced to the "players" on your rehabilitation team. You've learned that your family needs support in order to give you support. You've also learned some important questions to ask when choosing a rehabilitation facility. But there's still one element you need to understand before entering the world of rehabilitation. It's actually six elements in one, six arenas that are especially pertinent to SCI.

MOBILITY

The last thing Robert remembered was flying over the snow-covered rock on his skis. When he regained consciousness in the acute-care facility of a local hospital, he was in a state of panic. He couldn't move his legs. He had no sensations below his rib cage. He began to cry. Why couldn't he have been buried in the snow forever!

But that was several months ago. Robert is now in a quality rehabilitation facility where he is learning to use a wheelchair better than he'd ever learned to ski. With various types of therapy and treatment, he has realized that the wheelchair could have been his friend or his foe. He has chosen it as a friend, a very good friend. He has entered the wheelchair culture, forming new friendships and, at the same time, anticipating the day when he can go home to his family, to the house that is currently being made wheelchair accessible. He relishes the independence his wheelchair has given him. He is mobile once again. Robert may even ski again — sitting down!

Mobility is the number one arena in SCI. Accepting the fact that you cannot walk ever again, learning to handle a wheelchair, regaining strength and restoring balance, expecting and reaching a new-found independence though "seated" — these are the goals of mobility in rehabilitation.

BLADDER AND BOWEL

For Ruth, the most devastating result from her fall down the stairs was her inability to control her bladder and bowels. She had lost sensation below her waist and could not tell when she needed release. But, with good rehabilitation, Ruth learned that she could handle her new fact of life with a minimum of embarrassment or attention.

Bladder and bowel management helps SCI survivors learn new ways of functioning. In rehabilitation, you will learn that it is a very common result of SCI — and one that can be successfully handled. You will learn how to use unfamiliar equipment; you will learn how to adopt to a new way of life without sacrificing independence.

SEXUALITY

Sex had always been a major part of John's life. A bachelor in his late 30s, he enjoyed dating and never thought in a million years that he'd ever lose his drive. But that was before his car accident, when he had an injury to his T12 vertebra and not only had to learn how to use a wheelchair, manage his bladder and bowels, but also cope with the fact that he had lost the ability to perform sexually.

John started drinking to try to cover up his misery; he only felt worse. Luckily, with the proper rehabilitation, he learned to accept his situation. He learned how to give pleasure and find different modes of pleasure in return.

SPINAL CORDS

*"There are no hopeless situations; there are only men who
have grown hopeless about them."*

— Clare Boothe Luce

The sexual arena is an important focus of SCI rehabilitation. A good facility
will help treat sexual matters pertaining to fertility, performance, and ability.
The rehabilitation team will use understanding and sensitivity as well as
introduce equipment and methods that can help.

SKIN CARE

As far as Alice was concerned, skin care was something she read about in
magazines. It meant pampering at a spa and using creams and lotions to keep
crow's-feet at bay. But when she fell on the ice outside the grocery story,
smack on her spine, skin care took on a whole different meaning. Suddenly,
she had to watch out for pressure sores on her immobile skin; she had to be
careful of dryness and irritation that could lead to infection.

Skin care in SCI is critical. Because you may not be able to move your arms
or your legs, you can develop harmful pressure sores, which can lead to serious infections. A loss of sensation means that your skin can become very dry,
bruised, and irritated — without your feeling a thing. Good rehabilitation
always includes skin care therapy. You learn how to examine your own body
and change position to relieve pressure and prevent pressure sores.

RECOGNIZING THE RISK OF CERTAIN COMPLICATIONS

The words "autonomic dysreflexia" meant nothing to Billy. Neither did
"syringomyelia." A stockbroker by trade, Billy never gave the future a
thought. His great passion outside the floor was skydiving. One unfortunate
afternoon, his chute wouldn't open. Billy ended up a quadriplegic and these
unknown words became fraught with dangerous possibilities.

Spinal cord injury has many "spin-offs" in addition to immobilization and
a loss of sensation. Long-term paralysis and a continuous sedentary position
can result in elevated blood pressure — one of the first symptoms of a highly threatening condition called autonomic dysreflexia. *(See chapter eight for
more detail on autonomic dysreflexia.)*

Infections can abound in SCI. Bladder problems make urinary tract infections (UTIs) very much a reality if you are not careful. The build-up of urine
can also create serious infections throughout your system.

Cysts can also form in the spinal cord, which can fill with spinal fluid. This is a disease called syringomyelia.

Last but not least, there are the dangers of pneumonia and other respiratory ailments. If your breathing is compromised, you won't be able to cough efficiently. Fluids build up in the lungs.

These complications sound serious and they are serious, but they don't have to be life threatening. In a good rehabilitation facility, you will learn how to recognize the signs of these conditions. You will learn how to prevent infection and high blood pressure. You will learn how to take care of yourself in as independent a fashion as possible to avoid these all-too-real risks.

THE PSYCHOLOGICAL REALM

The number one psychological problem in spinal cord injury? The loss of self-esteem. Just ask Margot. She had been a vivacious, athletic woman in her 20s when a drunken driver forced her rented compact off the road. Now, slouched in a wheelchair, she barely has the energy to put on make-up or wash her hair. Who cares? No one would look at her anyway.

Wrong! Soon after Margot began seeing a psychologist at her rehabilitation hospital and began taking antidepressant medication, she learned that the loss of self-esteem was very common — but it didn't have to stick. She realized that she wasn't the only one who'd been given this twisted piece of fate. It was very difficult to accept, but, somewhere in the recesses of her mind, she knew that eventually she would have to accept her situation. She would have to go on.

SPINAL CORDS

A LESSON IN LIVING

Selena Morgan, an occupational therapist at HealthSouth Rehabilitation Institute of San Antonio, likes to tell this story:

She'd been working on a project for a new Alamo sports arena in downtown San Antonio when she realized that all the inexpensive tickets were designated for wheelchair users. It was simply assumed that they could not afford better seats. Although Selena immediately ensured that there were seats for all wheelchair users at all price ranges, she realized that this was a myth that was so ingrained in society that even she, an experienced therapist, hadn't seen it at first!

Unfortunately, many people believe that anyone in a wheelchair has a drop in income when, in reality, financial status usually doesn't change. "I have several wealthy patients," says Selena, "whose lifestyles haven't changed at all. Instead of sports cars, they simply drive souped-up vans!"

Margot is not alone. Depression, anger, grief, hopelessness, and helplessness are all feelings SCI survivors can feel after their accident. But with the right kind of rehabilitation, they learn acceptance. They learn, if necessary, how to deal with a new financial status; they learn how to cope with stress. They learn to go on and see their spinal cord injury not as an end, but as a second chance at life.

This, then, in brief, is the world of rehabilitation. It's time now to address the six critical arenas of SCI rehabilitation one by one, starting with mobility.

MOBILITY

"After the diving accident left me without the use of my legs, the one thing I knew, the words that kept going through my head, was to get back, to get back as soon as possible. And that meant learning how to move again, learning how to get around by myself. My wheelchair means self-respect."

– An L2-4 spinal cord injury
patient during a physical therapy
session at HealthSouth

Marissa never saw it coming. She was riding her bicycle, free as a bird, her helmet in place, when the car came barreling down the road. She swerved away from the vehicle just in time. But the quick right-left move made her lose her balance. She bounced over the rocky soil on the side of the road for a few seconds, then boom, fell down, her back smack in the middle of a huge rock, the bicycle on top of her. Something clicked. Marissa felt a sharp, piercing pain, then nothing. She could not move her legs.

Later, in the acute-care unit of her local hospital, Marissa and her parents learned that she had sustained a flexion injury to her spine, to the C7 vertebra in particular. Neurological damage began at C8; her chart read C7-8.

In other words, Marissa had almost complete control of her arms, her elbows, and her hands. She could breathe on her own; her diaphragm wasn't damaged. But Marissa could not move her legs; she could not move her torso; her ability to cough was poor. And if you asked her, she would have said she had no control — over herself, over life. Without her legs, without movement, without breathing strength, Marissa felt lost. She was bitter. To her, there was no future.

A TOOL FOR A NEW FUTURE: THE WHEELCHAIR

Ask anyone who has had a spinal cord injury and you will hear the same words over and over again: "I need to move...I need to get around my house...I want to get into town...I want to go to work...I need to move to be independent."

Movement. Mobility. This is one of the most crucial arenas for people suffering from spinal cord injury. Learning a new way of maneuvering around the environment, the world, can make all the difference between discovering a new future — or falling into despair.

It makes sense that physical therapy during the rehabilitation process concentrates on mobility, and one of the first places where mobility begins — and progresses — is with your wheelchair. Therapists know that getting you in a wheelchair, even if you cannot transfer to one from a chair or bed yourself, will immediately give you a sense of freedom.

Depending on the extent (location) of your spinal cord injury, your physical therapist will either recommend a wheelchair that is motorized or manually operated. You might also be taught how to use leg braces and orthotics to help you walk when you are not in your chair.

Paraplegics can be trained in the use of braces and canes if their legs are not completely paralyzed. A physical therapist will work on flexibility and strength-training exercises to keep joints supple and muscles toned. (Stretching and toning are important for anyone with a spinal cord injury, regardless of function. By keeping your muscles strong and properly stretched, you can avoid painful spasticity, or involuntary contractions of your muscles, and contractures, the actual shortening of muscles and joints that severely limit your range of motion, which determines your ability to move.)

SPINAL CORDS

TENNIS, ANYONE?

If you lived even a century ago, a spinal cord injury would have meant the end of a vital, energetic life. You'd most likely be bedridden, dependent, and obese, dreaming about those days on your bicycle. Not today! Thanks to advances in technology and science, people with SCI can participate in almost every sport the able-bodied do, just with a different style. You can ride a bike, plunge into the water for a swim or some scuba diving, throw a basketball in a hoop, ski down the slopes or behind a motorboat, hit a one-two in boxing, judo, or karate, skydive, play quad rugby, do some track and field, play table tennis, lift weights, and more. In fact, sports are so much a part of SCI survivors, both before and after their accidents, that there are wheelchair track meets held across the globe. Additionally, the Paralympic games coincide with the able-bodied Olympics and include the same competitions.

Marissa, like many other low quadriplegics, had capabilities similar to paraplegics. She had some movement in her arms, but she couldn't move her legs at all. For her, a wheelchair that could be manually propelled with the arms was the equipment of choice.

Although low quadriplegics, like Marissa, might be able use a manual wheelchair around the house, the majority of high quadriplegics cannot move their arms and need a motorized wheelchair. These weigh about 80 pounds and can move over 5 mph.

Your physical therapist might also recommend a combination of chairs, depending on your ability to propel your wheelchair, your endurance, and your lifestyle. For example, you might use a motorized wheelchair for school or the office so you can function more efficiently. But, to keep up your strength and endurance, you might want to use a manual wheelchair around the house.

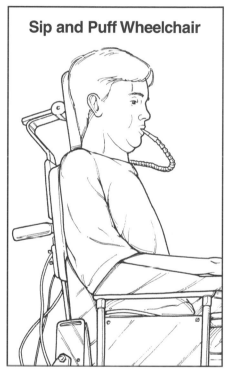

Sip and Puff Wheelchair

Do you have some movement in your hands and wrists? A motorized wheelchair that uses a <u>joystick</u> might be the right one for you.

Can you breathe on your own? If you are completely paralyzed, there is a motorized wheelchair called "<u>Sip</u> <u>and</u> <u>Puff</u>" that propels you along via air you blow into a straw.

Are you a high quadriplegic? If you are a C1-2, for example, and cannot breathe without a ventilator, you might be able to use a wheelchair with <u>headswitches</u>. A "cuplike" headrest with controls cradles your head; you use your head to put the wheelchair into action. Another choice: a wheelchair with <u>tongue</u> <u>control</u>. The keypad is literally placed on your palate. Other wheelchairs provide <u>chin</u> <u>control</u>; some will accommodate a portable ventilator.

SPINNING YOUR WHEELS

Think of the last time you bought a car. Most likely, you checked out the manufacturer. You determined the car's safety features, its durability, its comfort. You decided what you really needed — and what you could do without. Maybe you live in the country and you couldn't live without a Jeep for those

---

SPINAL CORDS

SCI MYTH #2:
EVERYONE WITH A SPINAL CORD INJURY HAS
TO USE A WHEELCHAIR

Wrong. Whether or not you use a wheelchair depends on where the spinal cord was injured. If you are a high quadriplegic, C3 and higher, you'll need a motorized wheelchair. Paraplegics and low quadriplegics can use a manual wheelchair, which are less expensive and easier to transport.

But many low paraplegics or patients with incomplete injuries are encouraged to walk, using braces and crutches. Although they still might use a wheelchair from time to time, the ability to stand and move helps their health immeasurably. If there's a possibility you can walk, as the commercial says, "Just do it!"

---

dirt roads. Or maybe you're a city person and a small car for those impossible parking spaces was more important.

Your wheelchair is like that car. It provides mobility. It symbolizes freedom. When you purchase or lease your wheelchair, you have to take into account the same factors as you would on that sporty number you want to testdrive. Here are some of the most important characteristics of a wheelchair you need to consider for the best, safest, and enduring ride of your life:

CONTROL: "I need to really hug the ground. I need to feel in control."

You have to feel secure in your wheelchair — and this means it provides the right amount of control you need for your specific mobility concerns. Perhaps you need speed to move through your office or across the street. Or maybe your house has many twists and turns; it's important for you to change direction smoothly. Whatever the scenario, you'll feel more secure in your wheelchair if you think of it as a vehicle to take you inside and bring you out, a matter-of-fact mode of transportation.

A motorized wheelchair also has to have some kind of microswitch, some kind of immediately accessible control unit. This can be a joystick, a "Sip and Puff," or the tongue control we talked about earlier in this chapter.

TIRES: "Don't tread on me. I want mine beneath me, in my tires."

Obviously, tires are a vital element in a working wheelchair. You need wheels that move, and that means good, durable tires. In the same way you'd choose tires for your new car, you want the best: a tire that holds up, that won't easily puncture or lose air. And, if you live in a climate where there's a lot of snow or sand, you'll want a tire with treads that can take it all in stride.

> # SPINAL CORDS
>
> ## *THINGS AREN'T ALWAYS AS THEY SEEM*
>
> *If you use a manual wheelchair, you might think that your arms are getting a great workout, that your range of motion in your upper body is in tiptop form. Not necessarily. The constant forward-leaning pushing can create rounded shoulders; you can start to droop. You need to do range-of-motion and strengthening exercises to move your shoulders in the opposite direction. Only then will your upper body have the total workout it needs for strength, balance, and healthy tone.*

You can get nonremovable, removable, or quick-release tires. Removable tires offer the most flexibility, quickly adjusting to your needs; they also make pushing and transfers simpler and more efficient. Further, they are less unsightly; you don't "hide" behind the wheel.

BRAKES: "I want to stop on a dime. Literally."

As much as you want to move, you want to stop when you want. You don't want your wheelchair to roll when you transfer to the bed. As with your car, your wheelchair brakes are vital for your safety. And, as with your car, they must be adjusted and tested periodically. Make sure you are able to use your brakes easily to stop your wheels, and that it isn't too difficult to engage them.

You'll find two main types of brakes on a wheelchair:

√ *High-mount brakes.* These are the most widely used brakes; they use a split clamp on the rear wheels at seat level to engage. Realignment is done by loosening the nut on the bottom of the clamp. However, if you are active, they can harm your hands.

√ *Low-mount brakes.* These look like scissors; they lock the wheels when you want to stop and move out of the way of the wheel when you release them. They are positioned on the bottom of the frame, below the seat, so that you will have to move slightly forward to engage. They are good for all sports.

√ *Hill climbers, or grade aids.* You can attach these to your high-mount brakes if you climb a lot of hills. They prevent you from rolling backward.

LEGRESTS AND FOOTRESTS: "Give me a place to put my feet up."

Let's face it. You are in your wheelchair for a good portion of the day. Your feet need to be comfortably placed at an angle that promotes circulation, prevents pressure sores, and reduces swelling. Your footrests should be aligned so that your knees are slightly higher than the hip. This is the optimum position for balance and less spasticity. There are four main types of legrests and footrests:

√ *Swing away footrests and legrests.* These are exactly as they sound. To disengage, the left and right rests "swing away" from each other. A variation for paraplegics: rigid frame wheelchairs with *footplates* that don't move, but are tucked back far enough for feet to be placed on the floor, and standing without any obstruction is possible.

√ *Elevating legrests.* These adjustable items allow you to move your legs further away from the chair, closer to you, or higher and lower. However, these legrests are rarely used except in problems with edema (swelling) or with motorized wheelchairs.

√ *Rigid adjustable footrests.* Rather than swing away from each other, these footrests are attached; you move them up or down for comfort. They are found on wheelchairs that do not fold. If you live an active life, these are the footrests — and the wheelchair — or you. They are lightweight, efficient, and help you move quickly; they also work well for quadriplegics and specially equipped vans. The adjustable footrests also protect your feet and add strength to the entire wheelchair.

√ *Folding footrests.* These are similar to the swing aways, but they are lighter. They flip up and are nonremovable. You'll find them on wheelchairs that fold.

ARMRESTS: *"A rest for the weary."*

Like your legs, your arms need a place to sit comfortably. Armrests are especially important if you use your hands to either brake or move your wheelchair; you need a position that will not add strain to your already working arm muscles. Look for adjustable height armrests if you use your hands. Arm locks help keep your limbs stable if you cannot move your upper body, or if your range of motion is minimal. Detachable armrests, either those that are completely removable or tubular arms that swing away, give you flexibility, making pushing your chair and transferring to your bed easier. Detachable armrests (as well as detachable legrests) are also necessary to facilitate getting in and out of a car or van. Although most paraplegics ultimately remove their armrests for good, they are necessary for those first few months when you are learning how to use a wheelchair.

HEADRESTS: *"Not for everyone."*

Not every model car has bucket seats. Similarly, not every wheelchair has headrests. They aren't necessary for paraplegics, who are usually positioned slightly forward in order to maneuver their wheelchair. However, if you are a quadriplegic, you will need a headrest; a proper seating system, with a

---

SPINAL CORDS

WHEELCHAIR SAFETY AND MAINTENANCE TIPS

- *If you have a motorized wheelchair, always keep a manual back-up just in case your batteries wear down unexpectedly — or if your van breaks down and you're left stranded!*
- *Add a seat belt to your standard equipment.*
- *Keep your seat clean! Use simple soap and water on a regular basis. Towel dry.*
- *Make sure your wheelchair has a warranty when you buy it, and bring it back to the shop for checkups once a year. It will save you the cost of repairs down the road.*
- *Spoke guards will prevent your fingers from getting caught in the wheel's spokes as well as protect the spokes themselves.*
- *Clothing guards act as side shields, protecting you from dirt, snow, water, and all the rest of nature's elements that might be thrown up by the wheels.*
- *Tire pressure should be checked regularly in order for your brakes to work at top performance.*
- *Check out the manufacturer Quickie's brand-new wheelchair. It is the first model that doesn't require tools to make adjustments. Cool!*

---

headrest, is needed for pressure relief. Your head also needs to be balanced for proper alignment and ventilator breathing. You'll find headrests in recliner models and motorized models with a Tilt-in-Space action.

SEATS AND CUSHIONS: "If I'm sitting all day, I need to be comfortable!"

You might already have the color and the fabric picked out, but unless your seat is comfortable, the most spectacular combo won't mean a thing. You'll be using your wheelchair almost all day long and it's crucial that your wheelchair's seat does all the right things: keep pressure sores at bay, align your body, provide balance, offer efficient energy, and make you feel at ease.

Let's start with position. Ideally, you should be able to sit in your chair with your back to the frame and your knees bent; your knees should be slightly higher than your hips to help provide trunk control. This position provides easier reaching, propelling, and turning. The seat cushion should be no wider than the chair frame. Your legs should fit comfortably along the bottom frame, ending with your feet solidly positioned on their footrests. (The footrests themselves will be smaller than your feet.)

Motorized wheelchairs can come with a Tilt-in-Space device; you are able to move (or tilt) back in your chair while staying exactly where you are in your seated position. This enables you to adjust your seat and frame to offer pressure relief without having to continually reposition yourself. The seat in a Tilt-in-Space remains at a 90-degree angle, which allows for better positioning and muscle tone than other chairs.

If you have a manual wheelchair, you can find pressure relief with special techniques. These "pressure reliefs" push up and move from side to side according to the instructions you feed an attached control panel. A reclining back, either motorized or manual, can also take off some pressure and add a comfort zone. But unlike a Tilt-in-Space, you may need to reposition your chair with each pressure relief adjustment.Wheelchair cushions come in three basic designs:

√ Roho. No, it's not a new fashion import. It's an air-inflated rubber cushion that provides the best protection from pressure sores and skin irritations. A Roho cushion is also great for balance; its surface of different-sized, contoured bubbles helps correct position and maintains your individual balance. The downside? If it is not inflated correctly, you'll sacrifice that balance. Roho cushions are also susceptible to air leaks and punctures. A hint: Keep a spare handy in case your Roho springs a leak.

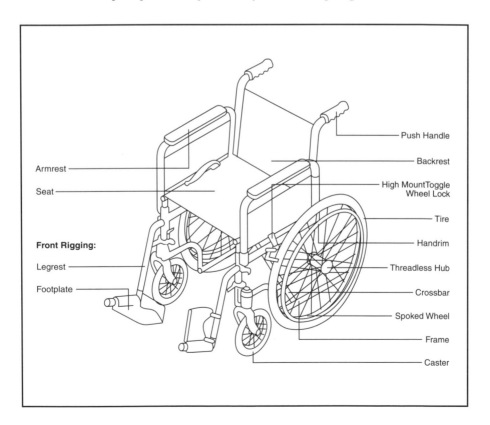

Armrest

Seat

Front Rigging:

Legrest

Footplate

Push Handle

Backrest

High MountToggle Wheel Lock

Tire

Handrim

Threadless Hub

Crossbar

Spoked Wheel

Frame

Caster

√ Gel. This cushion is filled with gelatinous material that is more similar to the dessert than the hair style aid. It provides much better body balance, but it is heavy.

√ Foam. The most versatile cushion of all. Foam can be shaped to your body; it's light and provides both balance and pressure relief. An added plus: It's the least expensive.

You can opt for a seat cover or not, although experts recommend you use the cover that comes with your gel cushion. Upholstery fabric is optional. Do you plan to use your wheelchair outside a lot? You might want to opt for a waterproof material. Is it cold in your neighborhood? You might opt for wool, leather, or sheepskin. Housebound? Maybe you'll want to opt for a bright color. Are you a high quadriplegic who'll be in your wheelchair more often than not? You'll want a durable, washable, and versatile material that will take you from a restaurant to the mall, from the supermarket to your job. Remember, as with any fabric, the more customized, the more the expense.

A TOTAL PHYSICAL WORKOUT

Although an education in the use and maintenance of your wheelchair is vital for any physical rehabilitation to succeed, it's not the only "course" you need to take. In order to graduate to physical independence with all your potential in place, you'll need to see your physical therapist for more mobility exercises. You'll need to:

• *Learn transferring* from wheelchair to bed, from bed to chair or toilet. Whether you can eventually transfer on your own or always with some help, it's important to know the basics. It's vital not only for independence and control, but to ensure pressure relief, proper circulation, and freedom from joint pain. The most important points? Always make sure your brakes are on and that your wheelchair is positioned for the most efficient transfer.

SPINAL CORDS

"Champions aren't made in gyms. Champions are made from something they have deep inside them — a desire, a dream, a vision. They have to have last-minute stamina, they have to be a little faster, they have to have the skill and the will. But the will must be stronger than the skill."

– Muhammad Ali, *The Greatest*

- *Perform range-of-motion exercises.* When you went through your day before your injury, chances are you were giving your joints, and the muscles, ligaments, and tendons that surround them, enough of a "workout" to ensure flexibility. But your SCI can create weakness, limiting the degree you can move your joints. The result? Less ability to do things for yourself. There's more: If your muscles are tight, your balance can go off kilter; you won't be able to clean yourself or position yourself during sex. You are more vulnerable to skin irritations and pressure sores as well as painful spasticity, cramping, and painful muscle shortening (contractures). But doing a series of range-of-motion exercises everyday can help ensure your muscles, joints, and tendons stay flexible.

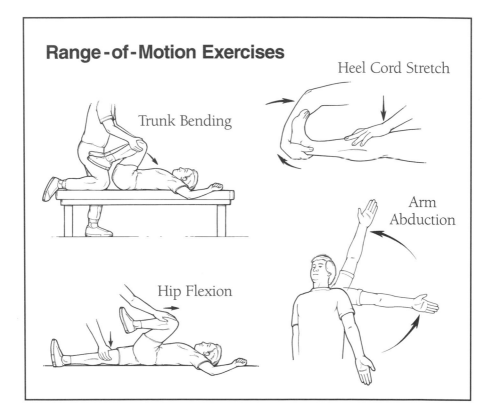

Range-of-Motion Exercises

Heel Cord Stretch

Trunk Bending

Arm Abduction

Hip Flexion

- *Practice prone positioning.* Unless you are on a ventilator, move (with or without help) from a sitting position to a prone position, straight on your stomach, several times a day. Wheelchair users run a high risk for tight, flexed hips and knees from sitting or lying on one side so much.
- *Help in the decision-making process.* You might be in excellent hands, but let your needs be known. If you can direct your care, explaining to your therapist where muscles are tight, when the best time of the day for prone

---

SPINAL CORDS

A PROPER FIT: A WHEELCHAIR CHECK LIST

Sitting in the right position in your wheelchair can go far in preventing pressure sores, contractures, spasticity, swallowing and respiratory problems. It can help you maneuver, become independent, and feel comfortable the whole time using it.

But it's easy to feel overwhelmed when you first get your chair and are bombarded with information on balance, pressure relief, and the whole gamut of wheelchair movement. "How do I know I'm getting the right chair? I'm not sure I can handle this." These are all anxieties we hear time and again. Don't worry. Take a deep breath and know that getting the facts will help you make an educated decision and give you the security you'll need that you've done everything right.

In that spirit of understanding, here are some tips to help you know you have the right fit:

- Your feet are flat on the footrests.
- Your elbows are comfortably bent on the armrests.
- Your thighs are parallel with your seat or slightly higher.
- Your knees are comfortably bent at the edge of the seat.
- You have a half-inch breathing room between your hips and the sides of the wheelchair.
- Your bottom is flush with the seat angle of your chair.
- You are sitting in a balanced position. This doesn't mean head up and stomach in, but rather a position where your knees are slightly high and bent and your head is slightly down. This provides better trunk control, reaching ability, and coordination. But make sure you keep up your strengthening exercises, particularly the muscles of the shoulders, girth, neck, and legs. And keep on pressure relieving!
- Your brakes, control panel, and on/off switches are easy to reach.
- You can maneuver easily in your chair and can stop when you have to.
- You feel comfortable! After all, you'll be in your chair for a large part of your day.

positioning is for you, how you can get more out of your range-of-motion exercises you'll be more in control of your own body and health — and you'll feel stronger and more motivated to go on!

- *Understand the signals your body is giving you to avoid contractures.* Your physical therapist will help you discover the cues that warn you of muscle shortening or spasticity before it becomes irreversible, and she can plan an exercise routine to meet your needs.
- *Become ambulatory if you are a low paraplegic.* Physical rehabilitation will include showing you how to stand, walk with braces, as well as with a new gait. You'll develop your muscles in your trunk, legs, and feet. Both quadriplegics and paraplegics can also benefit from stretches, pressure relief, and aided standing programs.

Mobility is a vital element in any successful spinal cord injury rehabilitation. But there are more arenas to explore, other rehabilitation roads to seek. Let's go to another important arena now, one that might feel humiliating, but is very, very common; one that, with rehabilitation, can give you a great sense of independence and control.

BLADDER AND BOWEL MANAGEMENT

"I confess. After my spinal cord injury, I thought about being able to walk. I thought about sex. But I never thought about going to the bathroom, that I'd have to relearn something so basic. It was a shock — but I wasn't alone."

– An 18-year-old skier who suffered a C7-8 injury

The injury had only happened a few weeks ago, but to Joshua it already seemed an eternity. At first, in the acute-care unit, he hadn't thought about anything but the pain. He couldn't move his legs, but his family kept telling him that it was temporary, that he would regain feeling once the shock of his football accident subsided. "Don't worry, dear," his mother would say. "You're going to be fine." She would then turn around, and even though she tried to hide it, Joshua knew she was crying.

There was always someone around: a doctor, a nurse, his mother or father. Everyone was always fluttering around him while he slept, on and off. He had no time to think; he didn't want to. His body was laid out in traction; he had to lie still. Tubes of fluids flowed in and out of his body. Machines bleeped and buzzed. His arms were weak; he found that his hands were shaped like claws when at rest; it seemed natural to keep them curled.

Joshua couldn't tell you when he first realized that his injury was more serious than what his family told him. He knew that he still couldn't move his legs; he knew enough about spinal cord injury to know that something like that had happened to him.

It was a nightmare come true for Joshua. But he didn't just have to learn to live with his paralyzed legs, his spastic arms. To his horror, Joshua realized that he couldn't control his bladder or his bowels. He had no urge to eliminate; he had no idea when he would "let go." Suddenly, what had been completely automatic, something he had done since he was 2 years old, had to be relearned.

Within another two weeks, Joshua was transferred to a rehabilitation hospital. There, he learned that bladder problems were common among SCI survivors. Even more comforting: There were ways to deal with it — and still have a normal life.

URINARY "TRACKS"

It's not something we think about — until we have the urge. And we can usually wait until we find a bathroom. Kids might have a harder time of it (especially when you're driving on a deserted stretch of highway), but once learned, elimination is as automatic as breathing or scratching an itch.

Basically, the foods and drink you consume turn into liquids as you swallow and digestion begins. By the time that now liquid apple or burger hits the small intestine, it's been divided into its smallest chemical components. Nutrients from these liquids are broken down, absorbed, and utilized by the

---

SPINAL CORDS

INCONTINENCE: IT'S MORE COMMON THAN YOU THINK

Believe it or not, approximately 12 million people suffer from a lack of bladder control — and many of them do not have a spinal cord injury. But if you do have an SCI, your situation is made more complicated — and not just because of your other conditions. Should you go for an external catheter or an indwelling? Which one causes the least risk of infection?

In addition to your doctor and your knowledgeable rehabilitation team, there are now two organizations where you can find a voice — without any embarrassment. These include:

Help for Incontinent People (HIP Inc.)
P.O. Box 544
Union, SC 29379
(803) 579-7900
Fax: (803) 579-7902
Toll free: (800) 252-3337

The Simon Foundation
P. O. Box 835-F
Wilmette, IL 60091
Toll free: (800) 23SIMON
www.simonfoundation.org

---

body as food. Waste materials are sent out of the gastrointestinal tract to the kidneys. More filtering takes place; toxic wastes are banished from the kidneys via tubes called ureters into the bladder.

Urine stays in the bladder until it gets full. A message is sent up to the brain: "I'm uncomfortable." The brain, in turn, sends down a response: "Find a bathroom fast." Once in position, the brain sends another message: "Relax." The urine leaves the bladder through a tube called the urethra. The muscles of the bladder contract. At the same time, the muscles of the urethra, the urethral sphincter, relax, letting the urine flow. Aahh....

Simple. Fast. And almost unconscious. But what if something goes wrong?

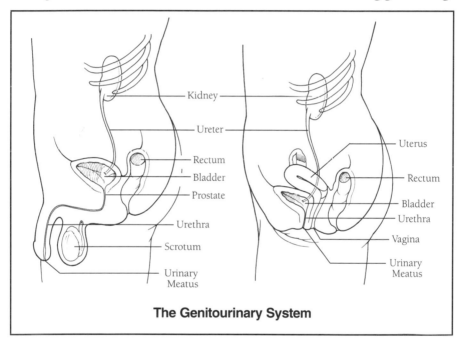

The Genitourinary System

BLADDER MATTER

As you now know, the spinal cord is a component of the nervous system, which includes the all-deciphering, all-knowing, decision-making brain. When something happens to the spinal cord, messages to and from the brain can get waylaid: They may fizzle out or never become activated. This is particularly true with the reflex actions of the bladder.

The bladder muscles contract at a signal from the reflex arc, located near the end of the spinal cord. As the bladder fills, the reflex action is to empty — regardless of where you are. If you'd been driving your car with a mug full of coffee inside you *before* your SCI, your brain would intercede. It would stop the reflex action; it would overrule the reflex arc and keep you full until you reached a bathroom. You might be uncomfortable, but you wouldn't be embarrassed.

But if your spinal cord injury occurred above the reflex arc, your brain can't intercede. It simply doesn't get the message. The reflex action will still be intact; your bladder will be able to empty. But you won't know when. This is called a spastic or reflex bladder.

If your spinal cord injury is low and has possibly damaged the reflex arc itself, your bladder becomes what we call "flaccid." In addition to the uninformed brain, you also have a reflex action that no longer works. You won't even know when your bladder will empty — you won't even know it's full.

SPINAL CORDS

SCI MYTH #3: PEOPLE WITH SPINAL CORD INJURY HAVE A GREATER RISK OF GETTING BLADDER CANCER

If you are an SCI survivor, it's understandable that you might be worried that your bladder problems can lead to infection — and cancer. But the reality is that although bladder cancer is more common in SCI survivors, the rate is still extremely low.

Among the normal population, approximately 1% of the population suffers from bladder cancer. Among SCI survivors? Only 3%.

Continue to seek your physician. Stick with your bladder management program. But don't worry needlessly.

FILLING THE VOID

A bladder that isn't functioning properly is not an insignificant problem. It is not merely a question of embarrassment. A malfunctioning bladder can have serious implications throughout your entire body. Perhaps your bladder empties, but not completely. Perhaps your bladder doesn't empty at all. The residual urine that is left in your bladder can pool and become stagnant like a forgotten pond. You can develop an infection. In fact, urinary tract infections (UTIs) are the most common complication among all spinal cord injury survivors.

But UTI is only part of the story. Some of the urine can back up into the kidneys, overloading and damaging them so they cannot do their waste-filtering job. Blood, filled with toxic waste, can be circulated throughout your system — with serious results.

A bladder program is essential to avoid these complications, and it is one of the first routines established at your rehabilitation center. In order to determine the extent of your bladder problems — as well as any progress you are making — your rehabilitation team might choose to do one or more of these diagnostic "elimination" tests during your stay:

"Elimination" Test #1: Urinalysis

This is one of the basics, one you've probably had every time you had a physical. You simply fill that little cup. A technician can determine your cellular and chemical make-up, make preliminary conclusions about blood cells in your urine (a sign of infection), possible diabetes, and more.

"Elimination" Test #2: Urine Culture

This is a more extensive procedure that might require placing a catheter in your bladder. Your specimen will be sent off to a laboratory where a culture will be "grown," determining if any bacteria are present. If your doctor suspects a urinary tract infection, she will also request a urine culture sensitivity; this will help decide which antibiotic will be most effective to treat the infection.

"Elimination" Test #3: Intravenous Pyelogram (IVP)

Don't be scared! This sounds much more imposing than it really is. An all-encompassing IVP is performed to see if the entire urinary system, including your kidneys, urethra, and bladder, is in working order, and, if not, where the problem lies. After a complete bowel elimination, you are injected with an iodine dye, which can be traced by an X-ray.

"Elimination" Test #4: Renal Scan

A clue: Whenever you see the word renal, the kidney won't be far behind. This test is another one that injects you — this time with a radioactive material that enables diagnosticians to analyze blood flow and function in the kidneys.

"Elimination" Test #5: Ultrasound

Like the sonar on submarines that depicted enemy ships, this device, placed on the skin, actually uses sound waves to create a picture. Sound bounces back and forth on the tissue walls, ultimately producing a depiction of an organ on a device very similar to a TV screen. Although no Kodak moment, these pictures show variations in measurement and shape, helping diagnosticians determine if you have kidney stones, tumors, or cysts in your kidneys, prostate, bladder, or uterus. Ultrasound will also pinpoint any residual urine you might have in your bladder after elimination.

"Elimination" Test #6: Cystourethrogram

No, you won't be asked to pronounce it, but you should be aware of this test. Another X-ray that utilizes dye (sent into the body via a catheter), the cystourethrogram helps diagnosticians analyze the bladder: its size, shape, and function. It is an important test for SCI survivors because the "C-gram" can determine if urine has backed up in the bladder and moved back to the kidneys. The result can be infection and a condition called reflux, which can severely damage the kidneys if not detected early enough.

"Elimination" Test #7: Cystometrogram

A cousin to the other unpronounceable test above, this one shows diagnosticians how your full bladder reacts to urine. Carbon dioxide or water, which mimics urine, is inserted into your bladder. The result? Your doctor can determine if you have a spastic bladder or a flaccid one. He can also see how much pressure builds up in your bladder before you need to void.

"Elimination" Test #8: Cystoscopy

Similar to a colonoscopy, a procedure that uses a snakelike device to probe your lower gastrointestinal tract, this test involves a lighted, flexible, camera-like catheter that travels through the urethra to the bladder to see firsthand if there are any problems. The images from the camera are displayed on a nearby screen. Don't worry. It's not as bad as it sounds!

"Elimination" Test #9: Urodynamics

This really isn't a single diagnostic test, but a term used to describe a series of tests that are analyzed and evaluated *together* to determine how you void your urine. It might include a cystoscopy, a cystometrogram, a cystourethrogram, and an IVP, among other tests that analyze your sphincter reflexes and your bladder's reaction to certain medications.

As you can see, bladder management is serious business. In order to find the best bladder program for you, some of these tests must be performed and re-evaluated throughout your life. They might get tedious, but your good health is worth it!

THE GREAT VOID: EFFICIENT ELIMINATION

Once your rehabilitation team knows the type of bladder problem you have, from a flaccid bladder to a spastic one, from kidney reflux to a urinary tract infection, a proper plan of action can be set. The main goal? Emptying the bladder without risk of infection and a minimum of fuss. Bladder problems can eventually improve in SCI, especially if you had an incomplete injury near the lower T or L/S regions, but you'll always most likely need some help.

Catheterization is usually the treatment of choice if you have little or no control. It is a remarkable piece of simple engineering. The plastic or rubber tube is inserted in the bladder to drain urine. Period.

Although the device itself is simple, there are various types of catheterization, one of which you'll most likely need after your spinal cord injury:

- *ICP* or intermittent catheterization program means exactly that: A catheter is placed in the bladder several times a day. There is a small tip at the end of the catheter that is inserted; the other end of the tube has a large opening. Urine flows out and is collected in a commode bag or collection device. ICP is one of the first steps toward retraining yourself in bladder management. Your rehabilitation team will help you learn how to do your own ICP at home, if necessary. You'll be surprised how easy and pain free this can be.

- A *Foley* or indwelling catheter may be necessary for high quadriplegics. It remains in the bladder at all times; it is changed every few weeks to help keep infections at bay. When a catheter is left inside, there is a greater chance for infection: *Cleanliness is crucial.* In Foleys and other indwelling catheters, the end of the tube that is inserted holds a small balloon. This is filled with water or saline solution to keep the catheter in place inside of the bladder. The other end is connected to an external collection bag.

- A *suprapubic catheter* is also left in the bladder. The device is placed directly into the bladder via a surgical incision in the abdomen. When your bladder is very weak, this might be the best catheter for you.

- *Bladder augmentation* can be an excellent choice if you are a woman who is a high quadriplegic with no urethra function. A catheter is surgically inserted through a hole in the abdomen (which can be covered with a patch). To help prevent leakage, a portion of the large intestine or the appendix may be used as an extra internal collection area near the hole; some surgeons may opt to enlarge the bladder instead.

- *External catheters* are condoms that fit over the penis; they are attached to a leg bag.

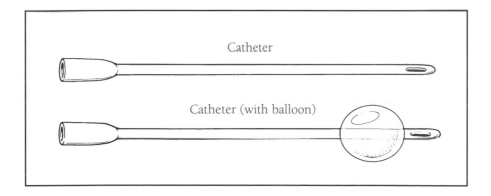

Catheter

Catheter (with balloon)

SPINAL CORDS

DISABLED PEOPLES' BILL OF RIGHTS AND DECLARATION OF INDEPENDENCE

We believe that all people should enjoy certain rights. Because people with disabilities have consistently been denied the right to fully participate in society as free and equal members, it is important to state and affirm these rights. All people should be able to enjoy those rights, regardless of race, creed, color, sex, religion, or disability.

1. *The right to live independent, active, and full lives.*
2. *The right to the equipment, assistance, and support services necessary for full productivity, provided in a way that promotes dignity and independence.*
3. *The right to an adequate income or wage, substantial enough to provide food, clothing, shelter, and other necessities of life.*
4. *The right to accessible, integrated, convenient, and affordable housing.*
5. *The right to quality physical and mental healthcare.*
6. *The right to training and employment without prejudice or stereotype.*
7. *The right to accessible transportation and freedom of movement.*
8. *The right to bear or adopt and raise children and have a family.*
9. *The right to a free and appropriate public education.*
10. *The right to participate in and benefit from entertainment and recreation.*
11. *The right of equal access to and use of all businesses, facilities, and activities in the community.*
12. *The right to communicate freely with all fellow citizens and those who provide services.*
13. *The right to a barrier-free environment.*
14. *The right to legal representation and full protection of all legal rights.*
15. *The right to determine one's own future and make one's own life choices.*
16. *The right of full access to all voting processes.*

RETRAINING SESSIONS

We might remember the slight embarrassment when we "slipped up," the slight dread if we mussed our sheets, but remembering exactly when we were "potty trained" is not something we'll be able to picture at the slightest nudge to our brain — even when we are training our own children.

That's why having to relearn bladder management after a spinal cord injury can feel so emotionally debilitating. But it's not. It's merely a physical function that has been disconnected. In most cases, you can retrain yourself to function without self-conscious embarrassment.

One of the goals of rehabilitation is to help you control bladder activity. It's one of the first things you'll learn because it is one of the first steps to independent living.

But there's more than the independence factor. There's the very real risk of

INTAKE/OUTPUT SHEET

DATE: _____

	INTAKE				OUTPUT		
TIME	ORAL	TUBE FEED	IV	TIME	VOIDED	ICP/FOLEY	VOMIT
7-3							
TOTAL:				TOTAL:			
TIME 11-7				TIME			
TOTAL:				TOTAL:			
TIME 11-7				TIME			
TOTAL				TOTAL			
24° TOT:				24° TOT:			

SPECIAL INSTRUCTIONS

RESTRICT FLUIDS   CC/DAY   FORCE FLUIDS   CC/DAY

Example of an intake and output sheet

infection, loss of muscle tone, and possible kidney stones if your bladder is not kept in check.

Because of the locale of your injury, you might never experience the "urge" again — or you may not be able to automatically control it. However, with training, you can learn a controlled *pattern* of elimination. You can learn when to go to the bathroom.

The most important element of bladder training is fluid balance, which doesn't mean equal time for drinking and elimination. You need to take in more than you put out in urine. Why? Bodily functions, such as sweating and even breathing, use some of the fluids you drink. If you don't take in *more* than you eventually release, you may end up dehydrated, which can be as dangerous to your health as a too full bladder.

Maintaining the right amounts of fluid also helps your bladder management program by helping you know when it's time to go. Drink between eight and 10 glasses of liquid a day, and try to avoid diuretic-like liquids, such as coffee and alcohol. Many rehabilitation centers provide charts to help you keep track of your daily intake and output or, as we call it, I & O.

FLACCID BLADDER IN TRAINING

Although by its very definition, a flaccid bladder cannot be controlled, you can still find some independence — and a decreased risk of infection and disease — through two maneuvers. (You will need a certain amount of hand function if one of these elimination programs is chosen.)

- To do the *Valsalva* maneuver, you should be sitting on the toilet. Hold your breath, push down, trying to use your abdominal muscles, as if you were going to move your bowels. Then relax. Continue this maneuver until your bladder has voided. **Note: Do not attempt this on your own. Because the Valsalva maneuver can increase heart rate and pressure in your head, you need to check with your physician to see if you are at risk. Some people are more sensitive to any stimulation.**
- You also need to be seated on the toilet to do *Credé's* maneuver. Here, you knead your fingers over your lower abdomen and bladder. After a few moments, relax. Then begin your kneading again. Continue until you have voided. **Again, please check with your physician before performing Credé's maneuver. If you have any bladder complications, it can make them worse.**

CLEANLINESS IS NEXT TO GODLINESS

The single most important thing you can do to prevent infection doesn't take a great deal of time. It doesn't cost a lot of money. And it isn't a complicated task you have to memorize and learn. It's called washing your hands.

That's it. If you remember to wash your hands before and after elimination, before and after removing your catheter, before and after cleaning your rinse bag, you can drastically reduce your risk of infection. This includes your caregiver as well. Washing your hands is just as important a rule for someone who is helping you with your bladder program.

Make sure your hands — and your catheters — are clean when you use them. Follow these tips:

1. Keep clean catheters separate from dirty ones. Use a plastic bag that is clearly marked.
2. Clean catheter with soap and water; follow with air drying. You can also use boiling water to ensure bacteria is killed.
3. Use an antibacterial wipe, such as Betadine, on your genitals.
4. Dry yourself carefully. Damp areas are prime real estate for bacteria to grow.
5. When in doubt, throw out old catheters. Always keep a fresh, new supply on hand.

THE REST OF THE STORY: BOWEL MANAGEMENT

Elimination is more than getting rid of the eight glasses of water a day you should be drinking. As we all know, the other normal human elimination function involves the bowel — and a different bodily system.

The gastrointestinal tract runs the whole length of the body. When you eat that apple or chocolate bar, saliva in the mouth begins to break it down and soften it for its journey down the gut. The food passes through the esophagus, the entrance to the stomach, and into the stomach itself. There, digestive action begins in earnest as that food is hit with stomach juices. Your apple, a complex carbohydrate, starts to break down into sugar, (the good kind your body needs for fuel) and your candy bar becomes fat, sugar, (the nonnutritive kind your body doesn't need) and a dollop of protein. Slowly this unrecognizable food travels to the small intestine where most of your digestive work takes place. Here, the food gets broken down even more, thanks to digestive juices, enzymes, and liver bile. The nutrients in the now unrecognizable apple or candy bar can then be sent to all parts of your body so hungry cells can eat (except that chocolate bar's fat goes to those ubiquitous fat cells for storage).

BULK ORDERS

Not every food you eat is used by the body. Waste cannot go to hungry cells; it would create infections. Where does it go? It goes into the large intestine where waste is stored, achieving bulk with undigested fiber and other by-products, until it leaves the end of the large intestine, the rectum, and out the anus as stool.

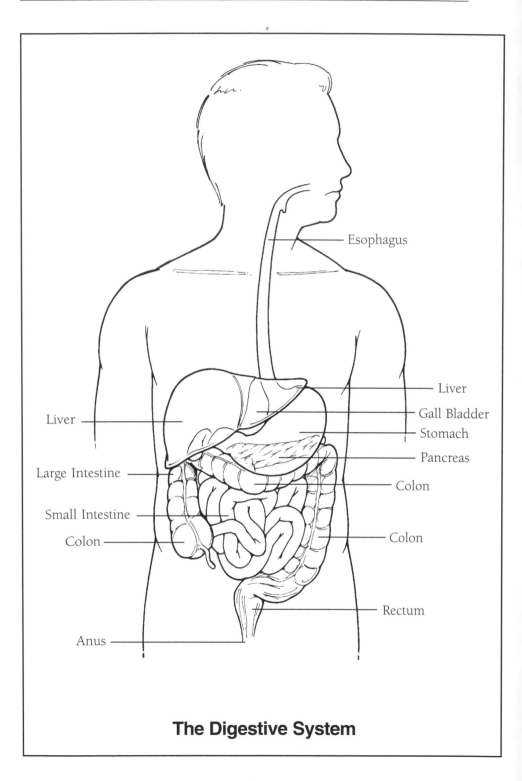

The Digestive System

SPINAL CORDS

IMPACTION: IT CAN HAPPEN TO YOU

You all know about constipation and diarrhea. But there is another condition that can cause diarrhea — and actually uses the same treatments as constipation. It's called impaction and it's a condition that occurs when stool is blocked in the large intestine.

Why can it cause diarrhea? Sometimes the only stool that can get past the blockage is soft or watery. diarrhea.

Try the same treatment for impaction as you'd use for constipation: high-fiber foods, psyllium seeds, exercise, and a regular bowel management routine. If you still have a problem, you might have to remove the stool by hand.

Still have a problem? It's vital you call your doctor to avoid any further complications.

In a perfect world, this process is also done without much thought (unless you've had a bout of food poisoning, an intestinal flu, or constipation). People develop routines; they have urges.

But after spinal cord injury, those reflexes that tell you to go to the bathroom may be lost. Like the reflex arc in a bladder condition, you cannot always tell when you have to eliminate. You might not be able to control it. You might not know if you have diarrhea or constipation. Some specifics:

- Slow, haphazard stool formation in the large intestine can occur after SCI.
- If you do not have feeling in your rectum, you will not have an urge to go.
- The sphincter muscle in the anus needs to relax in order for stool to pass out of your body. That same muscle needs to contract in order to contain a bowel movement at inappropriate times. SCI can affect your ability to control the sphincter muscle.
- If your injury is T12 or higher, you might not know when your rectum is full. Because your sphincter muscles are still intact, however, you might have a bowel movement without realizing it. This is called a *reflex bowel*.
- If your injury is T12 or lower, your reflex action can be damaged and your sphincter muscle will remain relaxed. This can cause impaction, constipation, and other conditions; it is called a *flaccid bowel*.

All is not lost. Like the bladder, bowel movements can be managed. You can learn how to control your bowel — and achieve more independence — with a program developed by your rehabilitation team.

YOUR BASIC BOWEL PROGRAM

The key word is planning. A regular schedule will help. You can help stimulate peristalsis (the movement of stools through the large intestine) with a suppository or by digitally manipulating the sphincter muscle. Wait 15 to 20 minutes and bear down. An abdominal binder can help tighten your lower abdominal muscles to better perform bowel management.

Everyone is different. Just as some people like to sit down on a toilet, magazine in hand, others like to get their bowel movements over with as quickly as possible. Similarly, some SCI survivors who are able to use a toilet prefer to sit down before putting in the suppository; others prefer waiting in bed until they are ready. Still others might like to sip a warm drink, like tea, while they work on their program. It's up to you. Whatever works within your functional ability. The important thing is that you have a regular program, one that you have worked out and *planned* with your rehabilitation team — and one that you can carry out on your own when you go home.

THINGS TO AVOID...

Here are a few things that can make it more difficult for you to maintain regular bowel management — and a few that can actually be dangerous:

√ *Check your medicine cabinet.* Certain medications can cause bowel problems. Talk to your doctor if you are taking any antidepressants, antianxiety medications, antacids, or cough and cold preparations. Some of these can cause constipation.

√ If you suffer from diarrhea, *watch out for spicy foods and caffeine. Be careful of overdoing laxatives* or bowel softeners.

√ *If you have constipation, try not to eat too many soft foods,* such as white breads, pasta, and other low-fiber products.

√ *Too much psychological and emotional stress* can play havoc with your bowels.

√ *Look out for beans, onions, peppers, sauerkraut, broccoli, apples, melon, Brussels sprouts, and cauliflower.* All of these fruits and vegetables can cause excess gas and intestinal bloating.

...AND THINGS TO EMBRACE

Here are some suggestions that can go far in keeping your bowel program on track and your body strong:

√ *Exercise* is important to incorporate into your new lifestyle. Range-of-motion exercises, upper-arm exercises, if possible, and stretching and using weights can help keep your bowels on a smooth, regular course.

√ *Eat a diet rich in fiber* to avoid constipation. These include whole-grain breads and cereals, vegetables, fruits, peanut butter, and lentil soup.

√ *Taking a psyllium seed product every day*, such as Metamucil, can help keep you regular.

√ *Keep to your program!* Losing an hour here, another hour there, will "confuse" your bowels. Sticking to your routine will help your body adjust to timely eliminations.

√ *Practice stress-reducing exercises.* Meditation, creative visualization, deep breathing — all these can help keep stress at bay. See your therapist. Join support groups. Talk. It helps, providing a necessary, crucial outlet — and hope.

√ *Cleanliness* is next to godliness, especially when it comes to SCI. Practice proper hygiene when you use your suppositories or perform digital stimulation. And *always wash your hands* after a "set."

Mobility. A regular bladder and bowel management program. You are getting closer...to getting back. But there are still a few important arenas to go. You'll find one of the most vital to your sense of well-being next: sexuality.

CHAPTER   SIX

SEXUALITY

"I was afraid of intimacy. I couldn't imagine having sex. But now I know I can have a sex life. Different, yes, but real — and close."

> – A 21-year-old college student who'd come to HealthSouth after a boating accident left him with a C6 spinal cord injury

Bill had had a spinal cord injury several months ago, a skiing accident that caused damage to his T10-11 vertebrae. He was able to move his arms; he had spent a long time in rehabilitation learning how to use a wheelchair, relearning bladder and bowel management. He'd returned to his job as a lawyer in a large Southwestern firm, and he'd even begun training for the Boston Marathon.

All in all, Bill seemed the ultimate success story of someone who'd suffered a SCI. He'd overcome many of his disadvantages; he'd learned how to cope with his new lifestyle. But there was one thing missing: a personal life.

Bill had joined a support group at his local rehabilitation hospital, a loose organization of single and divorced people with spinal cord injury. He made some new friends, but there wasn't any woman he was particularly attracted to.

Then he met Ruth, a new paralegal at his firm. She was able-bodied, but she didn't treat him with pity. She was forthright, kind, and at times she even seemed to flirt with him. Bill finally got up the courage and asked her out. Ruth said yes.

Bill went through several agonizing days before the Big Date. He hated the fact that here he was, a onetime powerful, big-time attorney, nervous about going out with someone of the opposite sex. He hated that he was filled with self-pity. He was so frustrated and fearful of rejection that he almost canceled the date.

But logic — and all those months of healthy rehabilitation — prevailed. Bill and Ruth went out, first to dinner and then to the movies. It was wonderful; she was everything he'd hoped she'd be. They had a lot in common.

Soon one date had turned into several; they'd become an item in the office. Their sexual activity had gone no further than some kissing, but both were ready for more. Bill explained that his SCI created some limitations; it didn't seem to bother Ruth.

But the worst happened. Bill had become so aroused that he'd forgotten to perform his bladder and bowel program before things got hot and heavy. He'd taken off his catheter and he ended up urinating on the bed.

Bill was so embarrassed that he couldn't speak. He was motionless. There was a pause. Ruth was the first to speak: "So. Where do you keep your sheets?"

She had turned a potentially negative experience into one that became more intimate. She'd treated Bill's condition with normalcy and rationality. No big deal.

And it wasn't.

In fact, in two weeks, Bill and Ruth are having a big wedding. The entire firm is invited — as is Bill's HealthSouth rehabilitation team.

MORE THAN FEELINGS

It's something that's difficult to accept. For many, it can sound like a death knell, a goodbye to pleasure. Unfortunately, the reality of SCI for many is the loss of sensation in the genital areas.

However, the loss of feeling, the inability to achieve orgasm, is not the only part of sexuality. It is a part, yes, — we won't pretend that it isn't. But it is not the *only* element of sex. There's the intimacy that comes with an embrace, the closeness, the tenderness, and the very real, heightened arousal. Indeed, many SCI survivors find that they can actually have a "psychic" orgasm, a feeling that is not unlike a real sexual experience.

In short, when you have a spinal cord injury, the same rules for "good sex" apply:

Good Sex Drive Rule #1: Feeling Good about Yourself

It's one of those credos: Feel good about yourself — and the world will feel good about you. The same applies to sex, with or without SCI. If you have a good perception of yourself, if you feel confident and secure, you will be able to enjoy yourself more — and offer more pleasure to your partner.

The fact is that the majority of people are slightly uncomfortable with a disability. They won't be attracted to you because of your injury — and they won't reject you because of it. But there will be some discomfort.

You can help put a potential friend at ease. If you feel good about yourself, he or she is more likely to feel good about you too.

SPINAL CORDS

A SEXUAL FACTORS QUIZ

Look over the following questions. See if any of them apply to you. If so, it's possible that you might be hindering your ability to enjoy a sexual experience. Talk to your physician or counselor — and your partner.

1. *Does your SCI change the traditional roles in the family? Turning you from a breadwinner to a homemaker? Does this make you feel dependent and unhappy?*
2. *Are you afraid of failing? Not only on the job or at home, but in the bedroom?*
3. *Are you pretending to be sick, hiding behind your SCI to avoid any possible confrontation or even physical pain?*
4. *Did you have a negative body image before your SCI? And now?*
5. *Did you have good sexual experiences before your SCI?*
6. *Do you have preconceived notions about sex, such as it's only for the young or that people will laugh at you if you show desire?*
7. *Are you depressed or anxious?*

Good Sex Drive Rule #2: Having the Ability to Communicate

Another component of a good sexual relationship is talk: the ability to talk about the things that bother you, that make you feel good, that make lovemaking more pleasant for the both of you. Obviously, with SCI, you will need to try different positions and different techniques that can satisfy both of you. The only way for this satisfaction to occur is through communication: talk.

Communication also means learning as much as you can about sexuality and spinal cord injury. It means talking to your rehabilitation team, to your friends in a support group, to your physician. You might lose some of the spontaneity of sex, but the anticipation that comes from planning can be exciting too!

Good Sex Drive Rule #3: Using All Your Senses

If you have SCI, you can compensate for physical maneuverability with your senses — and your imagination. Light candles. Create an atmosphere that is both relaxed and sensual. Remember, your senses can become heightened in areas other than your genitals. People with SCI have been able to "retrain" their bodies to feel arousal at other areas of the body: the face, the chest, the neck.

Good sex combines the sensual with the physical. In fact, without the sensual, the physical can be a turnoff — even if you have full use of all your limbs. Imagination can be very erotic.

Good Sex Drive Rule #4: Using Common Sense Doesn't Hurt

Although you don't want practicality to interfere with your romantic mood, SCI, as with any normal sexual encounter, requires a certain amount of "planning ahead." There are some basics you might want to perform before you begin an interlude:

- If you have a regular bowel and bladder program, perform it before you get comfortable.
- If you have an external catheter, remove it and either place it near the outside of your leg, or tape it to your abdominal area.
- Remove your catheter and collection bag. Make sure you've voided beforehand, and clean and wash your genitals.
- If you need assistance to get out of your chair and into a comfortable sexual position, have your partner — or an aide — help move you beforehand.
- Don't be afraid to tell your partner how he or she can best assist, including position and touch, for a maximum experience.

THE PHYSICAL FACTS OF SEX AND SCI

Some things never change. When you are sexually aroused, your blood pressure might increase, your heart rate will start to race, your breathing will become heavy, your skin will become flush and hypersensitive, and your muscles may contract — whether you have SCI or not. In fact, if you have spasticity, you might even be able to experience heightened sexual awareness!

But other areas of physical response may be changed forever, depending on:

- Where your injury has taken place
- Whether it is a complete or incomplete injury
- How long it's been since your injury — and how much rehabilitation you have had
- Whether or not you are taking certain medications.

SEXUAL CHANGES IN WOMEN WITH SCI

Unless you have a complete injury, it is possible that you will retain some feeling in your genital area. But sexual stimulation of the nerves endings in the clitoris can be altered. These nerve endings originate in the lower range of your spinal cord, from T12 through L2, and S1-4. If you have sustained

---

SPINAL CORDS

SCI MYTH #4: PEOPLE WITH SCI CANNOT HAVE CHILDREN

Wrong! In fact, a spinal cord injury does not usually affect a woman's fertility in any way. Half of the women who have an SCI never even skip a menstruation cycle, not even immediately after the injury; they remain fertile. If you do get pregnant, there are some special precautions you must take:

- *If your SCI is above T10, your labor and your delivery may be virtually painless — which can lead to a dangerous risk to you and your baby. From the 28th week on, frequent examinations are advised to ensure that you don't go into premature labor.*
- *Hospitalization is usually advised as you near your delivery date.*
- *Because of the risk of autonomic dysreflexia and its concurrent high blood pressure, keep all your doctor appointments — and be able to recognize symptoms of possible risk yourself. Your baby will thank you too! (See chapter eight.)*
- *You might need help during the delivery process if you cannot move your pelvic muscles. You might require a Cesarean mode of delivery.*
- *Men: Infertility is a possibility with SCI because of a lower ejaculation rate. If ejaculation is not possible, even after trying various techniques such as electroejaculation, vibratory stimulation to achieve ejaculation, and trial and error, there is always the possibility of adoption. (This is always an option, especially if you've tried fertility drugs, artificial insemination, and in vitro fertilization.)*

---

an SCI that is below these vertebrae, your genital area will be affected.

The good news is that with any loss, there is gain. In the same way people who lose their hearing might have heightened sight, you will experience more feeling in other areas of your body above your injury. Your breast area, for example, might become highly sensitized.

Your spinal cord injury might also result in a loss of lubrication. Without stimulation, your brain does not know it needs to send a message for more secretion in preparation for penetration. You can use lubricants to combat this problem. But stay away from simple Vaseline. It can become a "breeding ground" for bacteria and give you an infection.

You might not get your period for up to six months after your injury. But don't be alarmed. It's usually just the shock of the accident to your system. Most women find that their menstruation cycles become regular again before a year has passed.

SPINAL CORDS

"Disabled people are people, and people are people...virtually nobody is too disabled to derive some satisfaction and personal reinforcement from sex with a partner if possible, alone if necessary."

– Alex Comfort

SEXUAL CHANGES IN MEN WITH SCI

The nerves that control sensations and the flow of blood to your penis so that you can achieve an erection are, as in women, located in the lower area of the spinal cord, from T12 through L2 to the four sacral levels.

There are two types of erections:

- *Psychogenic erections,* which occur when your brain is able to deliver a message to your penile nerves, and...
- *Reflexogenic erections,* which are exactly as they sound: reflex actions that result from stimuli of the spinal cord itself. The brain is not involved. This type of erection is the most common in both the able-bodied and men with SCI. If you have had a complete injury, chances are you can still have a reflexogenic erection.

Fortunately, many survivors of incomplete SCI can achieve an erection with a little help. Quadriplegics can have an erection; the reflex action is intact. However, low paraplegics will not be able to have one because the nerves that create the reflex action are unavailable.

Some of the techniques developed to help men with SCI achieve an erection include:

- **Vasoactive Substances.** These materials can help enhance blood flow through your arteries to your penis and decrease the flow back through your veins. The result is an engorgement of blood — and an erection. You can actually inject these materials into your penis yourself with small needles, as directed by your physician. There are very few side effects with vasoactive substances. Talk to your doctor: New medications taken by mouth or inserted into the penis have been introduced into the market. Their use in people with a spinal cord injury is still being explored.
- **Vacuum Tumescence Constriction Therapy (VTCT).** This procedure involves a rigid tube placed over your penis, a pump that creates a vacuum, and a tight band around the base of your penis. The result? An erection.

- **Penile Prostheses.** These props come both semirigid and inflatable. Although they can help create an erection, prostheses can cause infection because they are surgically implanted.

Spasticity, too, plays a role. There's more chance of your achieving an erection if you are spastic than if you have a flaccid muscle condition.

Ejaculation, however, is another story. Because it is a complex result of a combination of various stimuli and responses, messages to and from the brain, reflexes and muscle contractions, ejaculation, more times than not, may be affected by your SCI.

One of the arenas that must be functioning in order for ejaculation to occur is your bladder; its neck must close so that semen can pass by without interfering with urination. If you have an SCI, it is possible that something called retrograde ejaculation may occur. Here, the bladder neck doesn't close and semen pushes through the bladder rather than through and out the urethra.

To help you ejaculate, you might want to try an over-the-counter, readily available vibrator; it can help stimulate ejaculation. However, a vibrator can also trigger autonomic dysreflexia, one of the risks of SCI (*see chapter eight*), and should be used only with caution. There are also electrical stimulating electrodes or probes that your physician can place in your rectum to help you ejaculate.

With a little forethought, knowledge, and understanding, sex, as with all the other arenas of SCI, can be a wonderful experience. Enjoy!

SKIN CARE

"Before my accident, I thought skin care was a vanity thing, something that cost money and reduced wrinkles. I know better now. Taking care of my skin has literally saved my life."

> – A 29-year-old woman who had a T10-11 SCI after falling down the icy steps of her front porch

The first few months after Meredith's sailing accident left her with an L1-2 spinal cord injury, she tried to do everything she was learning in rehabilitation. She worked on her physical therapy, learning how to transfer from chair to bed. She diligently performed her bladder and bowel program. Slowly, she felt herself getting stronger, better. She could even walk a few hundred yards with leg braces and crutches.

But enough was enough. Using a mirror to check her skin every day was something she rebelled against. Who had the time? There were so many more important things to learn, to change. She was receiving new vocational skills so that she could make the transfer from flight attendant to airline administrator. She was trying to make new friends and keep her relationship with her current boyfriend strong. When it came to these new experiences and learning how to walk and even go to the bathroom, skin care took a pretty low second place.

So Meredith merely nodded her head when her nurse mentioned her skin care routine. She told her team that she didn't need them to recheck her examination. Didn't they trust her?

This is the way it went — until a week before Meredith was ready for discharge and due to go home. It was when she'd transferred from her chair to the toilet that she first noticed the red sore on her thigh. She gasped. It was oozing, angry. Meredith was scared; she was afraid that her discharge would be delayed so she did the illogical, but impulsive, thing: She washed off the crusty ooze and denied that anything was wrong.

Two days later, the red, blistering sore had turned white. Now Meredith was really scared. She knew it was noticeable. It was only a matter of time until someone on the staff saw it; she knew she had to report it to her rehabilitation nurse.

It turned out that Meredith had a Stage 3 pressure sore, or ulcer, that could have been completely prevented if she had followed her skin care regime. Meredith's trip home was delayed another month while her ulcer healed. Dead tissue had to be removed; the sore had to be drained; the cavity had to be filled. The staff had to be on the lookout for dangerous infection that could spread to the organs of her body. But Meredith was considered lucky. The sore healed.

Today, she is scrupulous about her skin care regime. Meredith is careful to wash her hands and keep herself clean. She checks her body with a mirror every day — right after brushing her teeth.

MORE THAN SKIN DEEP

You never think of your skin as important, say, as your heart or liver. The integumentary system, as the skin is called in scientific terms, is never discussed among patients in the same serious breath as the circulatory system or the nervous system, for example.

However, in reality, the skin is the first vital organ the world sees. It is the fortress against invading bacteria and infection. It helps keep you cool in summer and warm in winter. It keeps all your bodily fluids and organs nurtured, maintained, and comfortable. Nerve endings, sweat glands, and oil glands all have a home in your skin.

But, when you have a spinal cord injury, your skin becomes even more important, and it plays an even greater role in your good health.

YOUR SKIN'S FUNCTIONS: NEW IMPLICATIONS FOR YOUR NEW WORLD

There are four basic areas, four "SkinScapes," that have added meaning if you have a spinal cord injury:

SkinScape #1: Protection, Protection, Protection

That special shield that skin offers in the able-bodied needs extra upkeep if you have a spinal cord injury. Depending on your level of injury, immobility is a greater factor. You aren't moving around as much; you are putting constant pressure on your butt, your thighs. Your legs no longer have the constant circulation of blood and fluids which movement provides.

The result of this immobility? Breaks, bruises, and tears in your skin you cannot feel. Irritations you might not know exist.

These irritations are called pressure sores, or skin ulcers. They can occur in

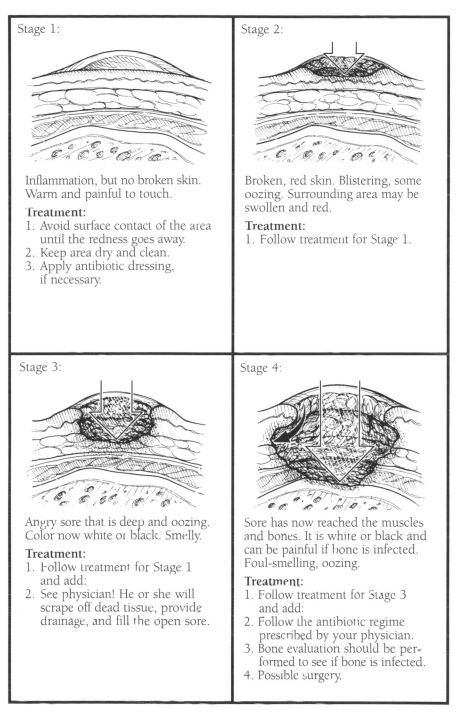

Stage 1:

Inflammation, but no broken skin. Warm and painful to touch.

Treatment:
1. Avoid surface contact of the area until the redness goes away.
2. Keep area dry and clean.
3. Apply antibiotic dressing, if necessary.

Stage 2:

Broken, red skin. Blistering, some oozing. Surrounding area may be swollen and red.

Treatment:
1. Follow treatment for Stage 1.

Stage 3:

Angry sore that is deep and oozing. Color now white or black. Smelly.

Treatment:
1. Follow treatment for Stage 1 and add:
2. See physician! He or she will scrape off dead tissue, provide drainage, and fill the open sore.

Stage 4:

Sore has now reached the muscles and bones. It is white or black and can be painful if bone is infected. Foul-smelling, oozing.

Treatment:
1. Follow treatment for Stage 3 and add:
2. Follow the antibiotic regime prescribed by your physician.
3. Bone evaluation should be performed to see if bone is infected.
4. Possible surgery.

Pressure Sore Stages

anyone who is bedridden or in one position for a period of time. But they can be particularly dangerous if you have a spinal cord injury. In fact, studies have shown that 62.5 % of all SCI patients get a pressure sore following their initial injury; 21.3% get two pressure sores and 10.3% get three.

The pressure sores vary in severity. Forty-six percent end up with the most common, and the least harmful, called Stage 1 pressure sores; 38.3% have Stage 2 pressure sores; 11.9% have Stage 3; and only 3.8% end up with Stage 4, the most dangerous pressure sores of all. By learning how to take care of your pressure sores with constant surveillance and by having an attentive rehabilitation staff, pressure sores may occur, but they need not be serious.

SkinScape #2: Feelings

All those nerve endings embedded deep within the layers of your skin, or dermis, have a purpose. They provide a warning for your brain to give out an all-points bulletin: "Keep that hot plate off your lap!" "It's freezing outside and your toes are getting numb!" "That rose bush you just wheeled past just stuck you with thorns. Ouch!"

If you have no feeling in your limbs, you won't just ignore the message. You won't hear it because no message exists. The impulses delivering the message can't travel up to the brain.

The result? Possible injury, burning, frostbite, or infection that you must watch out for. You must be vigilant and use your common sense: Even if you can't feel heat, you know that plate just came out of the oven and it's going to be hot. You know the weather is below freezing so you don heavy-duty socks and boots. You know that rose bushes have thorns, so you steer clear. Ditto for space heaters, campfires, and bags of ice.

SkinScape #3: The Great Regulator

No, it's not another Arnold Schwarzeneggar role. Your skin is the Great Temperature Gauge. Environmental stimuli get "under the skin"; the brain responds with a message; the skin either cools off or warms up. But, without feeling, your body won't adjust to changes in the environment. Most people with SCI don't sweat, shiver, or have goose bumps below their level of injury. In other words, when they are cold, they won't tremble or get goose bumps. When they are hot, their bodies won't find relief through sweating.

This same malfunctioning regulator may create excess sweating or shivering in some people above the level of injury. If you begin to sweat profusely — and it's not 110 degrees in the shade — call your doctor immediately. You might have a serious condition called autonomic dysreflexia. (See chapter eight.)

It's up to you to become your own "weatherperson," taking an environmental check during the four seasons.

SkinScape #4: Keep Those Fluids Coming!

One of the many studies conducted on airlines found that those cramped little seats in coach can be harmful to your health. Health practitioners advise passengers to make frequent "pit stops" while in flight, getting up and moving to the bathroom or simply up and down the aisle. Why? Fluids can pool in your legs, making your ankles swell and, if you're vulnerable, creating blood clots in your unmoving, stationary legs that travel up to your heart or lungs.

If these conditions can occur to passengers who normally have use of their legs, what would sitting all day in a wheelchair do? Plenty. If you sit in your chair most of the day, your blood and bodily fluids can "pool" in your legs, creating potentially dangerous swelling, or edema.

Worse, without movement, your blood doesn't get enough opportunity to circulate around your body. Consequently, your hungry cells can't get their "food" from circulating blood and they can die. The result are those ubiquitous pressure sores.

The good news about your skin and SCI is that many of the potential "SkinScape" problems can be avoided with a little knowledge and a little time.

SKIN FIRST

One of the most important things you can do for your skin — and one of the first items you'll learn to do in rehabilitation — is a daily inspection. Because pressure sores are so common among SCI survivors, you need to check various parts of your body every day. How? Easy. With a mirror — and

---

SPINAL CORDS

THINGS TO AVOID FOR GOOD SKIN CARE — AND GOOD HEALTH

Avoid:

- *Balancing frozen food in your lap. You won't even know when you get frostbite!*
- *Spilling hot food or drink.*
- *Smoking — for all the obvious reasons and one more: You can burn yourself without even realizing it!*
- *Going out in weather extremes without being properly dressed.*
- *Creating too much moisture in your groin area. Keep your catheter clean!*
- *Tight clothing. Pants, tops, shoes, and slacks that don't let your skin breathe can hinder circulation.*

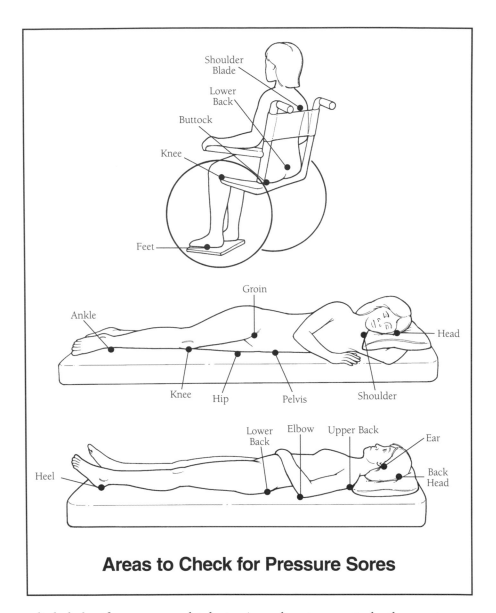

Areas to Check for Pressure Sores

a little help, if you are quadriplegic. According to one study, the most common areas on your body where pressure sores can proliferate one year after the injury include your:

√ Lower back — 20.5%

√ Buttocks — 18.3%

√ Heels — 16.6%

√ Hips — 12.4%

√ Ankles — 8.7%

√ Feet — 5.6%
√ Groin area — 4.5%
√ Knees — 3.6%
√ Elbows — 2.6%
√ Shoulders and upper back — 1.2%
√ Ribs — .4%
√ *And* unspecified miscellaneous areas, such as back of head, rim of ears, and upper arms — 4.7%

Nutrition is also critical to keep skin soft, smooth and pressure sore free. A well-balanced diet rich in lean meats, fruits and vegetables, and complex carbohydrates such as rice, sweet potatoes, and whole-grain cereals and breads, will help ensure that your body is getting the "food" it needs — which translates into healthy, toned skin and hearty circulation. Here are some other tips:
√ You might be trying to lose weight, but don't forget your fat! Essential fatty acids, found in fish and vegetable oils, help keep your skin moist.
√ Stay away from excess salt. Too much retains water, which can result in additional swelling, or edema.
√ Think water. Make sure you get the proper amounts of liquids for your bladder management program. This will not only help keep your bladder on an even keel, it will stop dehydration, which can harm your skin.
√ Avoid too much alcohol and caffeine. You might enjoy the taste, but they can lead to dehydration — not to mention anxiety and depression.
√ Take a multivitamin and mineral supplement with antioxidants every day. This will help ensure that you are getting the nutrients your body needs.

THE CLEANLINESS FACTOR

This is one of those SCI credos we can't say enough: Keep yourself clean! We've already seen how washing your hands before and after a bladder and bowel program can help keep infection at bay. Well, keeping your entire body clean can help keep infection away from your skin.

Think of it. Your skin's surface is over one square yard — a lot of territory where germs and bacteria can sneak around. If you have an open sore, a scratch, or simple dirty fingernails, you can be sure that bacteria are lurking, ready to enter through your skin and invade your body.

And speaking of dirty fingernails — and toenails: Keep nails trimmed and cleaned. Visit a podiatrist, if necessary. Short, blunt nails will ensure that you don't accidentally cut yourself or irritate your skin. It also keeps germs on a short "nail" leash.

SPINAL CORDS

SCI MYTH #5: PEOPLE WITH SCI GAIN A GREAT DEAL OF WEIGHT

Not necessarily. Statistics show that if people have a tendency to gain weight, they will, regardless of whether they smoke, drink, or use a wheelchair.

Of course, a sedentary lifestyle means that you are not burning as many calories as you might once have, especially if you were once an athlete.

More reality: For paraplegics, the ideal weight is 10 to 15 pounds less than for the able-bodied; quadriplegics need to weigh 15 to 20 pounds less. Why? There's more pressure on your body; gravity takes its toll. There's more of a risk of gall bladder disease, diabetes, and hypertension.

But, even with a less active life, you can still keep your weight off and within ideal bounds, and look and feel trim:

- *Exercise. Work on your upper-body strength. Have a "personal trainer" help you tone and stretch your legs. Swimming is the best choice for people with SCI. Let the laps begin!*
- *Try a new sport. Today, almost every sport has been redesigned for people with disabilities. You can do everything from horseback riding to sailing, skiing to basketball — and keep those calories burning strong!*
- *Eat a well-balanced diet, rich in fiber and low in fat. This doesn't have to mean deprivation. Think low-fat desserts and salad dressings. Pile on the fruits and vegetables. Enjoy hearty, whole-grain breads and cereals with skim or low-fat milk.*

Your best defense is not to be offensive: Stay clean. A daily shower or bath is a must. We suggest you wash your groin area twice a day. The moist, dark areas, where no air is circulating, are places germs love to roost. Use a warm washcloth, dry well, then powder with cornstarch. Another plus: You're also helping to keep your bladder and bowels infection free.

POSITIONS, PLEASE!

You can eat the right foods. You can do a mirror check every day. You can keep yourself clean. But unless you move around, those pressure sores are an ever-present danger. You need to keep your circulation going, too, to avoid swelling.

Positioning means turning, and it's something your rehabilitation team will help you learn during physical therapy. It might mean changing your position in bed from right to left. Or sleeping on your stomach instead of your back. It also means alternating your body alignment, using pillows to add and decrease pressure at various points on your body.

You should do a positioning exercise approximately every 15 minutes when you're awake and in your wheelchair. You'll learn these simple twists and turns from your physical therapist. They include:

√ Lifting your buttocks slightly and, holding on to the sides of your chair, leaning right to left.

√ Pushing up and slightly out of your chair.

√ Bending your chest forward and back.

√ Doing a "wheelie": Tilting your wheelchair back or using the recliner position.

√ Wiggling in your seat.

√ Proning: Getting into a prone position every day.

To get into the "swing" of positioning when you're in bed, try using an alarm clock, a wrist watch with a timer, or a beeper, set to go off after an hour or so, whenever you need to turn. Eventually, positioning will become second nature, just like your mirror checks or transferring from bed to chair.

Our rehabilitation journey is almost at an end. You now know the basics for proper skin care, wheelchair control, nutrition, sexuality, and bladder and bowel management. But there are still two arenas that are crucial for an up-to-the-minute, healthy, independent SCI survivor to know. Let's go to one of them now: recognizing the risk of certain complications.

RECOGNIZING THE RISK
OF CERTAIN COMPLICATIONS

"I have to watch out for problems more than the next guy. It's not some-
thing that makes me angry, just something I accept. I'm just really glad I'm
alive!"

— A 38-year-old man who suffered a T6-7 SCI after
a van swerved into the cab of his truck

The first time Ron experienced the symptoms of autonomic dysreflexia, he
was terrified. He didn't know what was happening to his body. All he knew
was that he woke up in the middle of the night, his eyes immediately blink-
ing open, his heart racing. He thought perhaps he had had a nightmare, but
he didn't have time to think about it. His head started to pound with a terrible ache; his face was sweating; he felt flushed and, at the same time, he had
awful chills.

"Help me!" he screamed into the night air. He wondered if he was having
a heart attack, or if he'd gone off the deep end and was having the worst panic
attack of his life. "Help!"

As his mother ran into his room, Ron noticed that his heart was beating
much slower; everything seemed slower. In fact, his vision was fuzzy, blurry;
he could barely see his mom.

Luckily, Ron's mother had learned that this might happen. The nurse at the
rehabilitation center had warned the entire family about autonomic dysreflexia. She knew that her son was having an "attack," a common occurrence
during rehabilitation stays.

Ron, 16 and vital, was having a difficult time adjusting to his new life after
a spring break car accident resulted in a T6 spinal cord injury. When it came
to learning independence, he did everything by the book. He wanted to be
free. So he practiced riding around in his wheelchair. He learned how to use
his catheter. He became a whiz at computer games and continued to do well
in school.

SPINAL CORDS

IF YOU'RE TIRED, YOU'RE NOT ALONE

More than half of the 300 SCI survivors interviewed in one British study suffered from fatigue. They were all under 60. Even more critical, these survivors were tired regardless of whether or not they were physically active and took care of their health.

But wait. Let's go a bit deeper. It turns out that these same people reported being tired three months earlier. In other words, their fatigue was always present. They were depressed, which affected their sense of well-being. They had more chronic pain. They didn't like to leave the house. They smoked.

Fatigue can be a complication of SCI. There is much more stress on your body. Every system has to work harder to go. But it doesn't have to be drastic. It doesn't have to be forever. Think positively. Ask your doctor about antidepressants and stay active. You can feel as if you've had eight full hours of sleep.

But he drew the line at certain, more sensitive areas of rehabilitation. Among them were the warning signs of autonomic dysreflexia. Didn't Ron have enough to worry about? Besides, he figured his mother would remember.

Ron had been having problems emptying his bladder and had just been fitted with an indwelling catheter that day at the rehabilitation outpatient clinic. Unbeknownst to him, it had twisted; his bladder was full. What would have been a signal of discomfort to him in the old days had turned into a life-threatening situation. Ron's body couldn't respond to pain in the more conventional ways. Instead of a rise and fall in blood pressure, there was a rise. Period. Ron's blood pressure continued to become elevated, and it was only his youth and his mother's foresight that saved him from having a stroke.

Ron's mother quickly inspected his body; she noticed the twisted catheter and untwisted it. As the urine emptied from Ron's bladder, his blood pressure started to lower; his headache eased. She also called the hospital; she wanted to be certain that Ron's blood pressure would go down to a normal range, and that he hadn't had any permanent damage to his body.

Autonomic dysreflexia is a complication in people, like Ron, with a spinal cord injury above or at T6. It is the way the body responds to pain when messages cannot be sent through the spinal cord. It can be one of the most critical complications of SCI, but it is by no means the only one.

LIVING SMART

Many of the complications that can arise in everyday life can be linked to genetic make-up, sensitivity to stress, the environment you inhabit, the lifestyle you share. If your father died of a heart attack, chances are you'd better have your blood pressure checked on a regular basis — and you should stay away from high-cholesterol foods. If you are fair, you are best to stay out of the sun and wear a thick sunblock whenever you do.

We think of these things as prudent, cautious, and smart. Why should it be any different *after* you suffer from a spinal cord injury?

The fact is that complications can arise when you have SCI. You do have to take precautions you might not have had to take before your injury. Like Ron and his mother, you have to be able to read the signs of any potential problem area so that you can handle a complication before it gets out of control. You can make a difference. You can make a complication easier to handle, if not simpler.

Let's go over the various complications that are prevalent in SCI, complications that can all be controlled with treatment, observation, and knowledge: [1]

The Combination Complication: High Blood Pressure, Excess Stress on Your Body, and Fatigue

Call them the triad, the enemies that when combined are a potent, silent problem — one that can lead to more serious complications such as autonomic dysreflexia (*see below*) and depression (*see chapter nine*). This "terrible trio" may physically stress your body and, in turn, compromise your immune system. The result? Once again, more serious complications.

What It Is & How You Get It:

High blood pressure, or hypertension, means that the force of the blood flowing through your arteries is too strong. Although you can't feel it, this force can weaken your artery walls. Your heart has to work harder to pump your blood through your body. Your blood is not circulating as efficiently as it should; small blood vessels cannot "handle" the flow of this forceful blood. The result if left unchecked? Heart attack, stroke, and accelerated atherosclerosis, or hardening of the arteries. High blood pressure can be genetic, but it can also be triggered by excess stress as well as situations more unique to SCI survivors: a full bladder, impaction, and autonomic dysreflexia. You have high blood pressure if your reading is anything over 140/90.

Excess stress on your body can also be a result of this high blood pressure, accelerated by the fact that muscles are tense, unused. If you have SCI, the reality is that you are going to sit in your wheelchair or lie prone in your

---

[1] *Pressure sores are the most common complication. See chapter seven on skin care for details and treatment.*

bed more than your active counterparts. This, too, adds stress, both physical and psychological.

Fatigue can have a psychological base. It can be a symptom of depression and a direct result of all that excess stress. Fatigue can also have a physical root: Your body has to work twice as hard to do what came automatically before your SCI. Breathing. Relieving your bladder. Getting from one room to another.

Treatment:

Hypertension can be controlled with medication. Your physician might have to try several different medications until he finds one that works. Then it's up to you to make sure you take your medication every day.

Exercise can help a body and soul under *stress*. And, believe it or not, exercise, not sleep, can usually wash away that tired feeling. Do your positioning exercises. Stretch. If you can, do upper-body exercises by pulling up and out of your wheelchair. If necessary, have someone help you stretch and massage your muscles.

But, because of the stress you put your body under every day, there are times when sleep is the solution. *Fatigue* might be your body saying, "Take a nap!"

Extra Hint:

Although the verdict is still out on definitive proof, taking a vitamin and mineral supplement may help your body fight off infection; it may help keep you strong and healthy. A long-term study of several thousand nurses in *The New England Journal of Medicine* found that 400 mcg of folic acid and 75 mg of vitamin B6 (both part of the vitamin B complex) substantially lowered the risk of heart attack by reducing the amount of histamine, a substance secreted by your body. Studies have also found that 400 IU (International Units) of vitamin E each day can also help reduce the risk of heart disease.

Antioxidants, such as vitamin C and vitamin E, have also been found to "gobble up" roaming free radicals, molecules that, if not destroyed, make your body's cells vulnerable to infection and premature aging.

You don't necessarily have to "pop a pill" to get your vitamins and minerals. Nutrition is critical for health, whether or not you have SCI. Eat a well-balanced diet, low in saturated fat and salt, high in fiber, with lots of fresh fruits and vegetables, and you can feel confident that you are getting the vitamins and minerals you need. In fact, everyone with a spinal cord injury should consult a dietitian.

SCI Public Enemy Number One: Autonomic Dysreflexia (AD)

AD is a condition unique to people with SCI. It can create dangerously high blood pressure and it's important to recognize its various symptoms:

- Pounding headache
- Chills
- Profuse sweating
- Flushing
- Stuffed up, congested nose
- Blurry vision

AD is particularly prevalent in people with spinal cord injuries above T6 (although it has been found in people with injuries as low as T10). Studies have found that approximately 85% of quadriplegics have had an episode of AD.

What Is It & How Do You Get It:

Autonomic dysreflexia is your body's attempt to deal with pain. Before your injury, a sharp, sudden pain would cause your blood pressure to rise. At the same time, the nerves would send a message to the brain via the spinal cord: "Ouch! I fell on my hip!" "Wow! That's hot." Your brain, in turn, would send two messages back down the spinal cord. One would ensure that you know, beyond a shadow of a doubt, that you hurt — and that you'd better take your finger off the stove. Your nerves would also get an automatic message, one born more of instinct than cognitive thought. This message would instruct your blood vessels to dilate, to open up. Your blood pressure would automatically lower back to normal.

But now, after your injury, your body's message relay system is off-balance. You can certainly still fall on your hip or touch a hot stove, but you might not feel any pain; your brain would not be able to register the "ouch." Further, although your blood pressure will still go up on impact, your brain won't be

---

SPINAL CORDS

THE ASHWORTH SCALE

How serious is your spasticity? Has it gotten any worse? One of the ways rehabilitation teams are able to diagnose your condition is with the help of the Ashworth scale. Here it is:

0 *No increase in tone. No spasticity present.*
1 *Slight increase in tone. There is a "catch" at the joint when the limb is either extended or curled.*
2 *More increase in tone, but joint is still moved easily.*
3 *A great deal of spasticity. Any movement is very difficult.*
4 *The affected area is immobile, caught in its state of spasticity, either rigidly out straight or rigidly curled.*

---

able to send a message down the spinal cord for the blood vessels to dilate. The nerves that would "handle" this message are blocked. The result? Blood pressure that stays dangerously high.

Treatment:

First things first: Sit up! Then stop, look, and listen. Some serious "spot checking" is vital to prevent an AD attack from getting worse — or preventing one from occurring. Always check your catheter to make sure that it isn't twisted; make sure your bladder isn't full. Check your rectum to ensure your AD attack isn't from constipation or impaction. Check your skin and body for signs of irritation or infection that might be triggering AD. (Don't forget to wash your hands before and after checking your bladder and bowels! It will go far toward preventing infection.)

Seek emergency aid immediately if you have any symptoms of AD, especially a pounding headache. And, once in the ER, don't let the attending physician send you home with a prescription for migraines. Make sure the ER knows about AD, its symptoms and dangers. A handy way to ensure you get the care you need? Carry a card that explains the symptoms of autonomic dysreflexia in your wallet. You can get a laminated wallet-sized card from the National Spinal Cord Injury Association (*see appendix C for full address and phone number*).

If you suddenly have symptoms of AD, your tendency might be to lie down. Don't! Remember: Sitting up will help ease your symptoms' severity. If you are lying down, raise the head of your bed.

Extra Hint:

Keep your fingernails well-groomed. Toenails need extra care too. You don't necessarily have to have someone sweep on red nail polish (especially you men!), but it helps to keep your toenails trimmed and cut straight across. Believe it or not, an ingrown toenail can cause pain and infection that can lead to autonomic dysreflexia.

The Other Common Complication: Spasticity

Forty years ago, spasticity was never used in the same sentence with spinal cord injury. It was a condition associated with cerebral palsy or stroke. The key problem was paralyzed muscles, not muscles that were too tight.

But today, with more and more SCI survivors, with more and more research, we now know that spasticity has a very real place in SCI. Along with fatigue, upper-body pain, and urinary tract infections, spasticity is another one of the most common complications of SCI.

What It Is & How You Get It:

Silent nerves along the spinal column do not just translate into limbs that won't move or bladders that won't function. Sometimes, these same disconnected nerves create the opposite effect: muscles that work too well. When a muscle contracts, the motion is a reflex action, an automatic response. If your nerves cannot receive a message from the brain that tells them to move that elbow back down, to uncurl that hand, to bend that straightened knee, to flex those pointed toes, the reflex motion remains. Muscles stay tight, contracted. If they remain in a rigid, straight form, you are in the midst of an extensor spasm. If your muscles remain bent or curled, you are having a flexor spasm.

Spasticity can also lead to contractures, a condition in which the tissues surrounding your muscles and joints become so tight that you cannot use the muscles you once could, such as in your arms, your shoulders, and your neck.

Although its roots are those malfunctioning spinal cord nerves, spasticity can be triggered by a variety of situations:

- *Pressure sores* irritating your skin.
- *A too full bladder* stretching the muscles in the area.
- *A full bowel* and its resulting constipation.
- *Paralysis after a spinal cord injury.* Your flaccid muscles might go through a period of spasticity several weeks after paralysis has taken hold. Physicians actually consider this spasticity good; it provides muscle tone to your once-flaccid muscles. It may go away by itself in time.

Treatment:

Although medications can work in reducing the pain and awkwardness of spasticity, they're not usually used right away. Sometimes spasticity will go away by itself. And sometimes, it can be used for good: helping you keep muscles toned and your bones strong, warning you that there is pain in a body area which you cannot feel, improving your sexual responses, and even helping you learn to walk with braces.

But, as with anything else in life, there is a downside to spasticity as well. Sometimes it can literally be a "pain in the neck." Prolonged spasms can create skin irritations and pressure sores. Spasticity can also interfere with your normal routines: driving your van, sleeping, and bladder and bowel control.

If spasticity is prolonged or interfering with your life, do not despair. There have been many inroads into treating your spasms and your rehabilitation team should be aware of them. These include:

√ *Antispasmodic medications.* Taken orally, these medicines will relax your tight muscles. Unfortunately, there are usually some side effects, including fatigue and dizziness. Your physician might have to try two or three different medicines until you find one that works well with a minimum of problems. Some examples include baclofen, zitanidine, and diazepam.

√ *Range-of-motion exercises and stretching.* Performing your exercises on a daily basis helps keep your muscles limber and also helps to avoid contractures. This "old-fashioned treatment" is more important than all the

---

SPINAL CORDS

SCI MYTH #6: PEOPLE WITH SCI DO NOT LIVE LONG, SUCCESSFUL LIVES

We won't pretend that there aren't days when you hate your new life, or that you would give anything to be on two feet again. But it's not all hopeless. Today, there are opportunities for people with SCI that weren't even dreamed about even 40 years ago. In fact, before World War II, most people who had a spinal cord injury died within weeks, usually from urinary tract infections, renal failure, pressure sores, or respiratory complications.

Today, with the help of advanced diagnostic tools, state-of-the-art medicines, and expert rehabilitation teams, people with SCI can look forward to many years of living well.

One of the predictors of a long, independent life? A good rehabilitation hospital. All the more reason to go to one that has an excellent record of getting people back to a meaningful life.

---

medicines and "high-tech" machines combined! *(See chapter four on mobility for these specific exercises.)*

√ *A standing program, or Grand Standing.* Weight-bearing, repetitive movements in an upright position help reduce spasticity and help stretch and strengthen the hips, knees, and ankles. Another benefit: By reducing the risk of osteoporosis, you are taking control.

√ *Splints and padding.* Using the "tools of the physical therapy trade" can help keep muscles straight, preventing them from curling rigidly out or in.

√ *Intrathecal baclofen (ITB).* If your spasms are intense and don't respond to oral medication and exercise, this may be for you. A titanium pump is implanted under your skin and liquid baclofen is dispersed at a controlled rate into your spinal cord. The result, a possible dramatic reduction in pain and spasm.

√ *Botulinum toxin.* Believe it or not, this antispasmodic, usually injected into the spot where the spasm occurs, is a derivative of botulism, the deadly food poison. However, here the substance does only good, smoothing out the tight, contracted muscles, but only in a limited number of specific muscles. Sold under the brand name Botox, it is considered so harmless that men and women have used it to smooth wrinkles on aging faces.

√ *Surgery.* If necessary, a neurosurgeon can perform a procedure on the spinal cord to reduce the impulses which are causing the reflex spasm.

Extra Hint:

Learning how to relax not only calms the soul, it can go far in reducing spasms. If you are less tense, your whole body loosens up — and that includes your muscles as well. Some ways to relax? Visual imagery. Deep breathing. Meditation.

The Complication with the Common Name: Calcium Imbalances — Heterotopic Ossification, Kidney Stones, and Osteoporosis

"Drink your milk." "Eat your broccoli." "Get at least 1,000 mg of calcium a day, regardless of age or sex." The truth is we never think of calcium as a bad thing. If anything, we always think of having too little calcium in our diet, not too much.

It is true, as anyone who reads the papers knows, that too little calcium absorbed by your body can create complications such as osteoporosis. But not as well-known is the fact that too much calcium can create kidney stones or, possibly, hormonal imbalance and heterotopic ossification.

In other words, SCI may create a calcium imbalance in your body which can result in a variety of complications. But there is good news: These complications can be managed with knowledge, care, and foresight.

What It Is & How You Get It:

After spinal cord injury, you can no longer use your bones the way you did. Perhaps you cannot walk. Move your arms. Your gait is much slower. Whatever the result of your injury, the decreased activity can make your muscles weak which, in turn, creates weakened, brittle bones, or *osteoporosis*. Although statistics are low on those people with SCI developing osteoporosis, the numbers may significantly increase as SCI survivors remain healthy and begin to age; it is found more in people who have flaccid muscle paralysis (rather than those with spastic muscles). The best defense for osteoporosis? Avoiding falls and other accidents that cause broken bones. Keep fractures and breaks at a minimum by learning everything you need to know about mobility (*see chapter four*) and, although it's a cliché, think before you act!

But after spinal cord injury, your body can react the opposite way: Too much calcium may float around your body. Combined with the change in your blood flow from decreased circulation and tears in weakened muscle and bone tissue, you might develop the strange-sounding *heterotopic ossification*. Studies have found that up to 53% of SCI survivors may develop this condition within three months of their injury. In this complication, new nuggets of bone actually grow between your muscles. Although this growth spurt usually doesn't last longer than two and a half to three years, it can limit whatever movement you might have in your joints. The area affected, usually the knees, elbows, thighs, and hips, can become swollen, red, and painful. You can also develop those contrary contractures, or shortening of muscles, which can threaten your independence and mobility.

In SCI, it's also possible that not enough calcium will be absorbed by the body. The excess calcium floating around your bloodstream can end up in your kidneys, creating painful *kidney stones*.

Treatment:

To help avoid *osteoporosis,* think exercise. *(See chapter four on mobility for exercise specifics.)* Do your stretches and range-of-motion exercises. Make sure you eat and drink enough calcium-rich foods: skim milk, broccoli, calcium-fortified orange juice, and dairy products. You might consider taking a calcium/magnesium supplement. The magnesium helps your body better absorb the calcium. You can find a variety of brands in your local pharmacy.

If you think you have heterotopic ossification, the first order of business is to have some tests done to ensure you don't have anything more serious, such as a bone tumor, an infection, or deep vein thrombosis. *(See below.)* These include:

√ *Alkaline phosphatase level testing.* If bone is growing in your body, the amount of this substance will be abnormally high.

√ *X-rays.* Yes, a simple X-ray can determine if you have any bone growth in your body.

√ *A bone scan* can provide a more detailed picture of your bones. It can detect early signs of heterotopic ossification.

The medicine Didronel has been found to help stunt the growth of extra bone.

You can help control *kidney stones* by eating less animal protein and sugar, both of which tend to make your urine more alkaline and susceptible to stone formation. Concentrate on fruits and vegetables. Maintain your bladder management program to prevent extra strain on the kidneys as well as possible sediment-rich urine backing up into the kidneys. (Maintaining your bladder program can also prevent urinary tract infections, a common complication in SCI. *(See chapter five on bladder and bowel management.)*

Extra Hint:

It's easier to prevent these conditions than control them once in place. Always perform your range-of-motion exercises gently and correctly. Eat a well-balanced diet, rich in fruits and vegetables. Avoid alcohol and caffeine, which can be "calcium leeches." And don't forget your positioning, turning and moving as your rehabilitation team taught you, to avoid pressure sores, which can trigger heterotopic ossification.

The Life-Threatening Complication:
Deep Vein Thrombosis (DVT)

Your blood needs to circulate smoothly and efficiently through your arteries in order to provide oxygen, or "food," for hungry cells; through your veins to carry waste off to the always-filtering liver and kidneys; and through *all* your blood vessels to maintain a clean, clear environment for "a good run" both coming and going. The very nature of SCI means that blood is not circulating briskly through your body, which may create a dangerous condition: deep vein thrombosis.

What Is It & How Do You Get It:

It's a fact: Blood has a tendency to clot if it's not pumping efficiently through your body. This situation can occur from stroke, hypertension — or spinal cord injury. If you've lost feeling in your legs, your muscles will not be moving the way they once did; they can't help pump the blood up, down, and around your legs. The result may be a blood clot. If it stays in the veins of your legs, it's called a thrombus. This situation is dangerous because a thrombus can easily turn into an embolus, a blood clot that breaks free of the vein wall and travels up...to your lungs. When a clot travels to your lungs, it is called a pulmonary embolus, which has been found in approximately 3.8% of SCI survivors.

If the clot breaks free, it can be serious and you need to get medical help fast! Here are some of the warning signs:

√ A sudden warmth in your legs, especially in your calf muscles.
√ Swelling and redness in your legs, especially your calf.
√ Tenderness in your legs by the veins, if you already have sensation.
√ Pain in your calf when your ankle is stretched.
√ A sudden, rapid heartbeat.
√ A sudden, intense fever.
√ Shortness of breath.
√ Tightness in your chest.
√ A sudden, violent coughing spell.

Treatment:

It cannot be repeated often enough. If you suspect DVT, call your doctor immediately, especially if you experience any shortness of breath and tightness in your chest. You will most likely be given an anticoagulant medication to break up the blood clot and prevent others from forming. While you are being treated, you will need to stay in bed for a few days. Do not perform your range-of-motion exercises. Wait until the crisis has passed.

Extra Hint:

DVT can mimic heterotopic ossification. Make sure your physician performs heterotopic ossification tests to rule it out.

A Complication You May Share with Dolphins: Breathing Problems

Dolphins do not breathe automatically. They learn from the moment they are born to remember to breathe. Even when they sleep, a section of their brain is awake, reminding them to breathe in and out.

Human beings have the luxury of automatic breathing; we do not have to think about it unless something happens to our respiratory system. A high level spinal cord injury can hinder that automatic breathing.

What It Is & How Do You Get It:

A spinal cord injury above C5 can paralyze the diaphragm, the major breathing muscle, at least temporarily. You will need a ventilator to help you breathe. *(See the next chapter on miscellaneous matters for information on ventilators.)*

An SCI above T1 can also prevent the intercostals, the muscles that sit between your ribs, from doing their work — helping you to breathe deeply as well as cough.

An injury above T12 may make your abdominal muscles weak, which can hinder your ability to clear your throat or cough when you have a cold.

SCI also leaves you more susceptible to infection — like pneumonia. You might have a respiratory complication if you:

√ Have shortness of breath

√ Start breathing rapidly

√ Get a sudden, pounding headache

√ Are feeling very tired

√ Have a fever

√ Have nasal or chest congestion

Treatment:

The best policy is prevention. Here's an obvious one: Don't smoke! If you need a ventilator, follow your respiratory therapist's instructions diligently. Perform your breathing exercises to strengthen muscles, allow more air to enter your lungs, and keep your lungs clear.

If you catch a cold, don't let it get worse. Call your physician and take whatever medicine is prescribed. Do your breathing exercises a few more times a day. Do some quad coughing exercises as instructed by your respiratory therapist: While a loved one or caregiver pushes in your stomach, cough. Repeat several times. A hot shower may help loosen mucus in your chest and throat.

SPINAL CORDS

"Strong hope is a much greater stimulant of life than any single realized joy could be."

– Friedrich Nietzsche

Extra Hint:
Try this easy breathing exercise: Take in as deep a breath as you can. Hold it for a count of three, then exhale. Repeat up to 10 times. This will help keep your lungs clear and your muscles strong. You can also use a "blow bottle." You breathe into a straw that leads to a small ball floating in air. As you breathe, you'll be able to see firsthand how much air is displaced with your breath. You can visually judge from day to day, week to week, how strong your breathing is becoming.

If you have weak abdominal muscles as a result of your injury, try an abdominal binder. It literally holds your stomach in, giving you "muscle power." Your ribs are kept in place; your breath improves and you can cough more efficiently. But a word of caution: Abdominal binders aren't for everyone. They can cause skin problems and you'll ultimately need more assistance in daily care.

A Common Problem for Both SCI Survivors and the Able-Bodied: Gallstones

A poor diet makes for a sluggish digestive tract. Unfortunately, SCI survivors have to be more disciplined in keeping their systems strong and healthy — and that includes the gut. This means that you might not be able to "get away with" as much fat and rich food as you once did.

What It Is & How Do You Get It:
Like kidney stones, gallstones are tiny crystals. But, instead of calcium, gallstones are made up of cholesterol. The hard-working liver makes both cholesterol, which is stored in the tiny gallbladder, and bile. The bile helps in digestion, breaking up food. Cholesterol is not only ingested, but also created from some of the foods you eat. When you eat fatty foods, an imbalance is created. The liver makes too much cholesterol — and too little bile. The result? Tiny deposits of cholesterol stored in the gallbladder.

You can go your whole life without knowing you have gallstones. In fact, many people do. But sometimes those little stones find their way to the duct that connects the gallbladder to the small intestine, creating spasms of pain and nausea. This can be particularly debilitating in SCI survivors. Studies have found that three times as many people with SCI have gallbladder disease than the able-bodied.

Treatment:
As always, the best treatment for gallstones is prevention. Try to limit the amount of fat you eat, including: saturated fats, like butter and coconut oil; animal protein, including marbleized steaks, sausage, and pork; and desserts rich in cream and butter. The less fat you eat, the less cholesterol your liver will produce. If your pain is acute, laproscopic surgery can be performed to remove the stones.

Extra Hint:
Too little fat can also create gallstones. The liver has less work to do and, consequently, produces less bile — which means that there's less bile to break down cholesterol. Once again, you have an excess of cholesterol stored in your gallbladder. The best solution is to eat some fat every day, but make sure it's of the nonsaturated variety, such as canola oil, olive oil, and safflower oil. Eat fish instead of reaching for that burger: It contains omega-3 fish oil, which not only produces "good" fat to keep skin healthy and hair glossy, but keeps your body "heart healthy." Studies have found that eating fish five times a week substantially reduced the risk of heart attacks.

The Complication with the Complicated Name: *Syringomyelia*

Syringomyelia can be present from birth or can occur after a spinal cord injury. You can develop it whether or not you have a complete or incomplete injury.

What It Is & How You Get It:
Basically, syringomyelia is a cyst filled with spinal fluid that forms within the spinal cord. As it fills, it can create more and more pressure on your spinal cord nerves, creating damage and wreaking havoc on your body. You can become more spastic. You can lose any sensation you might have. You can become at greater risk of getting autonomic dysreflexia. You can have more pain. Worse, if the cyst develops above your injury, it can make your SCI worse. Suddenly, you have symptoms, say, of a T5 injury, even though your injury occurred at T10. The worst part of syringomyelia? It can move into the brainstem.

Treatment:
Early diagnosis is critical to prevent further neurological damage. An MRI can clearly and painlessly show if there are any cysts in your spinal cord. If

95

one is present, it can be treated surgically. A tube is inserted into the cyst; the spinal fluid is drained away.

Extra Hint:

Don't wait if you feel you are not functioning as well as you once did. If you are feeling worse, get help! If you wait too long the neurological damage can be permanent — even with surgical intervention. Your best bet is to have an MRI if you experience the slightest change in neurological function. Can you still feel hot and cold with your fingers? Has your blood pressure gone up? Are you having more and more muscle spasms? Don't wait to see if they go away. Call your doctor. A good physician will be glad you did.

We've now covered most of the special arenas that make up the world of spinal cord injury. But there is still one place where we have not yet gone: the mind.

THE PSYCHOLOGICAL REALM

"When I first had my accident, it was who am I? Now it's what am I going to do next!"

– An 18-year-old athlete who survived a
snowboarding accident with a T4-5 SCI

When Mark came to HealthSouth, he'd just come from the acute-care unit of his local hospital. Homecoming had always been a big deal at his college and, as a newly minted freshman, Mark was ready to party. But as designated driver, Mark stuck to soft drinks and juice. Later, he and his friends were driving around the local streets, laughing, shouting at each other, the music turned up loud. They didn't see the driver heading the wrong way down the one-way street. It was a head-on collision. Ironically, Mark had been completely sober; the man driving the other car had been legally drunk. Mark was left with a sprained ankle, a few broken ribs — and a T11 vertebral fracture and spinal cord injury. He was the only one hurt that night.

His sprains and bruises healed well; Mark had been an athlete, a burgeoning quarterback, and in the prime of health. But his mind was not healing as well. He was understandably depressed, angry, and confused.

But if his rehabilitation was going to work, Mark had to have the right motivation. He had to have a positive attitude. The entire rehabilitation team had to help him get back — to the happy, kind, helpful Mark he'd once been.

One of the therapists suggested that Mark keep a journal, to write his thoughts down as a form of catharsis, to help him come to terms with what happened to him. Hesitatingly, slowly, he began. Soon the words rushed out.

"It's a Saturday and if I was back in college, I'd be going to practice. But I'm not. I'm sitting by the window in my room at a hospital and I am looking out at the lawn. It's flat, green. That's how I feel, flat. I want to get out of this wheelchair and crash through the window. I want to leap out onto that flat, green lawn and run. I want to run as fast as I can until I am so out of breath, I fall. I want to move. I want my legs to ache, to feel tired. I want to be myself again. I want to run, that's all. I just want to run. I'd give anything, anything, to be able to run."

Mark was in trouble. He couldn't get past his injury, his pain.

And there's no mistaking that pain. We could sugar-coat the entire process, offering you "psychobabble" about how you'll get better, that there's a whole new world just waiting for you, but it will only fall on deaf ears. Like Mark, you want to run and you can't. Period.

But, within three months, Mark started to get better. He began to see the possibilities that existed for him. He began to re-examine the things that were once important to him — and what was important to him now. He made new friends; he found himself reflecting on the world around him, on subjects that were once alien to him. In short, Mark began to grow.

It wasn't a miracle. It didn't happen overnight. But it did happen. And it can happen to you, despite how you might now feel about your spinal cord injury.

THE CRUELEST BLOW OF ALL

You know you are the same person. You know that you still love burgers and pasta. You can still balance your checkbook, work a computer, and laugh at a good joke. Your brain was not hurt, just your spinal cord.

But there lies a harsh irony. This same consciousness, this same level of intelligence that maintains your essence also reminds you, every day, every minute, that you cannot walk or move your arms or perhaps even breathe on your own.

Even worse, the people around you — your family, your loved ones, your colleagues, even people you barely know — don't seem to treat you the same way. They don't seem to think you are the same. It's as if they can't get past the wheelchair. Perhaps they'll talk louder to you, treating you as if you were mentally impaired. Worse, they might be solicitous, trying to help you as if you were a child. They might mean well, but their pity shines through.

In short, if you or someone you love has had a spinal cord injury, you know that one of its most frustrating — and cruelest — aspects is the fact that your personality is still intact, but your independence feels as if it's flown away, never to return.

You're still the same, but you are not.

Picture this scenario: Suddenly, you cannot move your bowels or manage your bladder. You can't walk. You can't get dressed by yourself, something that took minutes in your "old life." You can't even enjoy sex the way you once did.

Worse, you may not be able to do the job you once held down. Money becomes tight. This adds to your already mounting stress level. Perhaps you start to drink to ease the pain. You take drugs to self-medicate, which, in turn, creates infection and physical complications. You are in more pain. You are confused. You begin to drink more or take more drugs.

SPINAL CORDS

A PSYCHOLOGICAL ADJUSTMENT WORKSHEET

Answer these questions as truthfully as you can. They can help bring your world in focus and stop you from feeling completely overwhelmed and lost. Show it to someone on your rehabilitation team. Discuss it with people you trust.

When I first learned about my condition and all of its complications, I felt

_____

This is what I did to cope: _____

My greatest strength has been: _____

These people helped me: _____

The hardest part of this was/is/will be _____

I'm proud of my ability to _____

The changes in my activities are _____

The changes in my attitudes toward myself are _____

About my life in general are _____

About my body are _____

My fears about my spinal cord injury are _____

My thoughts and feelings about social/sexual/recreational/employment/ relationships: _____

What I have today that I didn't have before my spinal cord injury

_____

—Wanda Trojanoski, University of Rochester, Strong Memorial Hospital Rehabilitation Unit, *Spinal Cord Injury Manual*, Rochester, N.Y.: 1986. Revised: 1994.

Maybe your emotions get the better of you. You lose control more often, lashing out in anger at strangers or those you love. You become obsessed with your relationships, needy and as emotionally dependent as you believe you are physically.

It's frustrating. Your self-esteem is at a low ebb. You begin to spiral down into a profound depression.

STOP!

It doesn't have to be this way.

"I DIDN'T CALL UP A DEPARTMENT STORE AND ORDER THIS"

There's a saying we use with our new SCI patients: "It's not like you called up a department store and ordered a winter coat and a spinal cord injury." You didn't want it. And there is no way you would pick it out from a catalog and order one sent by express mail. But it's here: You have a spinal cord injury.

That realization is a difficult one to face. But face it you must if you will ever find relief. If you will be open to rehabilitation. If you will ever get back into the world.

Unfortunately, along with this sobering realization is another one, just as difficult, but one that is equally important:

Although there are a lot of people who are ready and willing to lend a helping hand, when the chips are down, it's you. You have to be the driving force. You have to find the perseverance, the determination, and the hope to help yourself.

It's tough. It's hard. But before you decide to rip this book up and throw it away, remember that accepting these facts is the first step towards mental health and psychological adjustment.

MAKING THE CHOICE: THE SECOND STEP

Once the emergency has passed, the diagnoses made, the rehabilitation program spelled out, and the all-important realizations made, you are left with two choices:

Choice #1: "Poor me, woe is me, there is no one worse off than me": Playing the Victim

Obviously, this is not the choice a good rehabilitation center wants you to make, but it is one that, consciously or unconsciously, is chosen time and time again.

A possible result?

√ *Alcoholism and substance abuse.* Research has placed the number of alcoholics and substance abusers among the disabled at 7 million. A study done at a Baltimore spinal cord treatment center found that 65% of its patients had a substance abuse problem within six months of their accident. More sobering news: A California branch of the Department of Veterans Affairs found that 75% of their members had a substance abuse problem *at the time of their accident.*

√ *Violence.* You may be angry at some point after your spinal cord injury; it's a healthy sign of acceptance. But, for some, this anger is so global, so fraught with frustration and stress that it becomes unmanageable. Not only do some SCI survivors lash out at inappropriate times, such as in a restaurant or at a party, but they can ultimately lose those people — spouses, lovers, and friends — who were initially there to help, creating even more hopelessness, rage, and psychic pain.

√ *Profound depression.* At least 11 million Americans suffer from depression — and many of them do not have SCI. It makes sense that a spinal cord injury will create a sense of hopelessness and helplessness. SCI survivors, usually vibrant, healthy, youthful people, find it difficult to have high self-esteem at first. Self-esteem is tied up with body image. But self-esteem can be redefined over time. Real, permanent self esteem comes from:

1. *The three "A's":* Affection, attention, and acceptance from others.
2. *A sense of competence.* A job well-done can go far to help *anyone's* self-esteem.
3. *A moral standard.* Whether religious, ethical, or moral, having a belief system and sticking to it will simply make you feel good about yourself.
4. *A feeling of power.* Through rehabilitation, you can learn self-control. You can learn how to take care of yourself — and influence others. You can find an inner strength, which means that you know, deep inside where it counts, that you can influence your fate. You have some say. You are still you.

√ *Dependency — on a person and your relationship.* If you are beginning to feel depressed, your self-esteem and self-control nonexistent, you begin to look outside yourself for help. You can begin to feel desperate, totally dependent on someone else for your safety and love. The result? A caregiver who is exhausted and frustrated too. A person who might be thinking of leaving. In fact, it is this fear of dependency that makes many SCI survivors struggle for hours to get dressed, to try and independently perform their daily functions before starting their day. This not only makes them exhausted before they've even gone out the door, but helps sustain

---

SPINAL CORDS

ARE YOU DEPRESSED?

Take a few moments and read over this quiz. If any of the statements ring true, you may be suffering — needlessly — from depression. See your physician. He or she can help ease your pain.
 1. *I'm eating too little — or too much.*
 2. *I'm not sleeping at all.*
 3. *I can't get out of bed in the morning.*
 4. *My head is full of "shoulds" and "what ifs." I can't stop thinking about what I did, and continue to do, wrong.*
 5. *I can't concentrate on my rehabilitation routines.*
 6. *I'm tired all the time.*
 7. *People are telling me how cranky I am. I know I'm really irritable, but I can't stop it.*
 8. *I have a very short fuse lately. Anything can set off a rage.*
 9. *I am filled with a sense of hopelessness.*
10. *I think about killing myself. (If you answer yes to this last statement, call your physician immediately. You need help fast!)*

---

those negative feelings of frustration and hopelessness. A better bet: hiring a personal assistant who can help you with your daily routines. You'll leave fresher, happier — and with a good night's sleep. Remember: You would hire someone to, say, fix your roof or play music at your wedding, so why not someone to help you maintain a feeling of self-control and getting things done, which is the core of independent thought.

√ *Extreme stress and anxiety.* Contrary to popular belief, stress can be good for you. It's how you cope with it that causes problems. Sometimes a bit of stress propels you to finish a job, to do your range-of-motion exercises without fail. But stress can also overwhelm you, creating inertia and that old enemy, depression. This type of stress is most common after a life-altering event — such as a spinal cord injury. Remember these three "R's":
1. *Recognize the stress.* Are you too exhausted to get out of bed? Are you constantly fighting with your husband or wife? Have you lost your job or find you can no longer make ends meet?
2. *Receive help* — from your rehabilitation team. Chances are, they'll recognize the signs before you and will make sure you get the help you need.

3. *Relax* — with prescribed antianxiety medication, deep breathing exercises, and meditation.

Believe it or not, these particular situations are not carved in stone. You don't have to be a victim. There is good news: another choice, another path you can take. It's the one that will make you grow, change you for the better, and help you live an independent, full life.

Choice #2: "I have a spinal cord injury. I can't change it — no matter how hard I try. So. Let's get on with life!" or Accepting, Looking Ahead, and Seeing a Future

Life is bittersweet. It contains the good with the bad, the winning with the losing. It's a fact of life that we will feel loss at one time or another. Grief is universal. Approximately 30 years ago, Dr. Elisabeth Kubler-Ross presented her landmark six emotional stages a person must go through when tragedy strikes before they can get on with life.

Although she was talking about her six stages within the context of terminal illness, they can apply to spinal cord injury. You may go through all these stages, some of these stages, or only one or two, before this second choice can become a reality:

Stage #1: Denial. Shock has a purpose. If you felt the full impact of your spinal cord injury all at once, you would feel totally overwhelmed. Your brain protects you with denial. "Sure," you tell yourself. "I'll walk again. This is just a temporary problem that will go away in no time."

Stage #2: Anger. Anger is an appropriate response to a tragedy. Remember, you didn't pick out a spinal cord injury from a catalog. Of course you're angry. Dr. Albert Ellis coined a phrase that keeps many of us in a holding pattern, spinal cord injury survivors or not. "I *should* all over myself." Think about it. "I should do this. I should have done that." These thoughts can make you dizzy, frustrated, and terribly, terribly angry with yourself and the

---

SPINAL CORDS

"It is an amazing tribute to the flexibility and magnificence of the human spirit that so many people whose lives are thus devastated survive and function at the level of physical and social independence which most cord injured people achieve."

— G.W. Holmann, 1975

---

world. Forget what you *should* have done — the past is the past. You can still do something about tomorrow — starting today. Try to understand why you are angry. Accept it and work through it. But don't punish yourself for what *should* have been.

Stage #3: Bargaining. This is the stage where negotiations become critical, the time when we try to "reason with our God" to change the way things are. "I'll be a better person if you'll only give me use of my legs again." "I'll never go skiing again if you'll make me better." You need to pray for a miracle. Once you realize that you are going to have to live with and adjust to your spinal cord injury, you'll be able to move on. It's the only way to come to terms with your life.

Stage #4: Depression. Yes, it's true. You need to feel that hopeless and helpless feeling. You need to feel sorry for yourself. After all, you'd have to be superhuman in order to feel fine after a spinal cord injury. It hurts. Everything hurts. Your life is different. You have to mourn. You have to feel bad. Don't worry. You'll come out of it — especially with a good rehabilitation team ready and willing to help. There is a light at the end of the tunnel.

Stage #5: Acceptance. At last! You've cajoled and bargained. You've gotten angry. You've felt so depressed you thought you'd never smile again. But, slowly, carefully, you've come up from the ashes, your mind intact. Your rational self knows that things are different, that they will never be the same. You accept that and are ready to make the healthy choice: getting back.

Stage #6: Hope. Believe it or not, with your newfound acceptance comes something you thought you'd lost forever: hope. For a new, good life. For the promise that you have. For life.

These six stages are not a *fait accompli*. Not everyone goes through each of these stages or goes through them in the same order, especially people with spinal cord injury. But, hopefully, you will experience many of these emotions during your rehabilitation. They are necessary in order for you to be motivated enough to have, hold, and maintain a new life.

A good rehabilitation hospital will help you get back to your life with an experienced, professional staff and a sound, consistent program. Some of the psychological tools they'll use include:

√ *Education.* In knowledge there is strength. And nowhere is this more important than in getting on with your life after a spinal cord injury. You need to learn new skills for your new life. How to use a wheelchair or braces. How to meet new people. How to nurture old friends who don't know how to respond to you. How to continue in your career of choice. Armed with education, you can enter your brave, new world with dignity, empowerment, and a sense of independence. From being out of control to being back in the driver's seat — once again controlling your own destiny.

√ *Medication.* Although your depression might have been triggered by the emotional impact of your injury, it may also have a biological component. Your attempt to adjust to your new life and your feelings of dependency and despondency pile on the stress, which can affect the subtle chemical pathways in your brain. To help ease your pain and keep a positive attitude in place, your physician may recommend an antidepressant medication. These may include Prozac, Zoloft, Paxil, or amitriptyline. You may have more success with one over another, and you might have to do some "trial-and-error" work with your doctor. If your stress also makes you nervous, your physician may also prescribe an antianxiety medication, such as Valium, Xanax, Ativan, and Klonopin. One note: Both antidepressants and antianxiety medications may cause such side effects as dizziness, fatigue, and foggy thinking. You must be closely monitored while you are on these medications.

√ *Therapy.* Yes, that good old-fashioned talk can help you learn the tools you need to cope with your new life. A trained counselor in a one-on-one session can help guide you through the six stages of grief. A psychologist can also provide a necessary outlet for you without fear; you can say anything you are feeling without possible repercussion. Today, most counselors are eclectic. They may use some behavior modification techniques, classic psychology, and common sense logic. The main component in therapy that helps ensure its success is the relationship you maintain with your counselor. You might have to "shop around" until

---

SPINAL CORDS

SCI MYTH #7: PEOPLE WITH SPINAL CORD INJURY END UP DIVORCED OR IN BAD MARRIAGES

Wrong. In reality, the number of divorces in marriages where one of the partners has SCI is equal to the number of divorces in able-bodied marriages! In other words, if you have a solid marriage or relationship before your injury, chances are it will continue to be strong. True, your partner will need some advice and education from your rehabilitation team; a therapist can help your loved one deal with his or her own grief and confusion. But, the fact remains that few able-bodied leave.

Even better news: There are fewer divorces in postinjury marriages than in able-bodied "I do's."

---

you find someone you trust, someone you like, someone you can relate to. Although you lose the intimacy of a one-on-one talk, group therapy and support groups have other benefits. They provide a "mirror" to the world at large, proving you are not alone. Another person with SCI will understand what you are going through better than anyone else. You can help each other find that inner strength to face the world. Support groups can also help you cope with alcohol and substance abuse.

The world of psychological adjustment has many answers and many opportunities for help once you make the choice to get on with your life. The more help you receive, the better you feel and the better rehabilitation works — and the faster you get back. Start now!

MISCELLANEOUS MATTERS

"I used to be so confused about everything. There was so much to keep track of! But, like learning a new language or sewing a dress, it's become second nature. And so has my independence!"

— A 21-year-old schoolteacher who skidded her
car on black ice, resulting in a T10-11 SCI

Remi wasn't afraid of using a computer. He was a whiz on the Internet, and he could type 120 wpm on his keyboard. He wasn't afraid of his remote control; he'd click the buttons faster than a fade-out on the television screen. Nor was he afraid of aiming his wheelchair down a hall, once he got the hang of it, or "stroll" into town to shop.

But FES? No way.

It wasn't the name that scared him. In rehabilitation, Remi learned that it wasn't some kind of exotic hat. FES stands for Functional Electrical Stimulation, and it's used in many rehabilitation centers. It is also used as a component in a program called the ERGYS system.

All these strange names were intimidating to Remi. They sounded way too sci-fi for him to feel comfortable. Worse, the theory behind FES and ERGYS sounded like something straight from "The X-Files": Electrical impulses stimulate the muscles of your arms and legs to make them stronger.

Too weird. Especially because Remi, like many of the other people at his rehabilitation center, couldn't use his legs. He was a paraplegic and could handle it just fine now, thank you. What did he need ERGYS for? What was all the fuss about FES?

The machinery, too, was daunting — equipment with computers and electrodes that seemed to grow larger every time he looked at it.

But two months later, Remi was ready to become a FES spokesperson. His physical therapist had gotten him to try one of the machines, and he found, like the Lifecycles he'd used before his accident, that he could turn the wheels. The computerized machine helped give his legs the message to move; he was bicycling! He felt invigorated. Free.

It wasn't some kind of mumbo jumbo. Nor was it a miracle. It was simply science at its best at work. Electrical impulses in various tempos were sent out to Remi's quadriceps, hamstrings, and gluteal muscles. Shocked into action, these muscles contracted. The rhythm of the contractions pedaled the stationary bike.

Why FES? Even the Food and Drug Administration recognizes that the ERGYS system for fitness helps reduce muscle spasm, atrophy, pressure sores, urinary tract infections, and edema. (FES itself is a general term to cover many different types of muscle stimulators, including the ERGYS system.)

There's more. ERGYS also improves blood circulation to the legs, range-of-motion potential, bone density, and bowel function. But it's not for everyone. If you have frequent bouts of autonomic dysreflexia, bone fractures, dislocated joints, or osteoporosis, ERGYS might be hazardous to your health. But even if you are a prime candidate to get on and ride, it's important to avoid unrealistic expectations. ERGYS and the FES system can only do so much. And remember to go slow! It takes time to feel comfortable with any new exercise equipment.

Fortunately, Remi took to ERGYS as if he'd always ridden a stationary bike. Backed by its benefits and his own positive results, Remi could not stay afraid for long. Today, he has his own unit set up in the workout room in his house. He calls it the FES health club. "All that's missing is a sauna. Now that would be nice."

Maybe you're not like Remi. Maybe the idea of electrical stimulation doesn't make you shiver. Perhaps you were ready to get on the bicycle as soon as it was introduced in your rehabilitation program.

But perhaps there's something else that confuses or overwhelms you, some miscellaneous matter about your spinal cord injury rehabilitation that you just can't fathom. We've included some of the more common "extras" below. We hope they help clear things up.

COVERING THE BASICS

Function is more than form. It can mean the difference between independence of any kind and dependency. It can mean the difference between self-control (and self-esteem) and depression. That's why your rehabilitation team spends so much time on bladder and bowel programs *(See chapter five for specifics.)* Once you've learned your program, including how to use your catheter and how to time your bowel movements, it becomes second nature. Taboos are lifted and you can begin to feel like a "person" again. Your program becomes as routine as brushing your teeth or making your lunch.

The same goes for mobility. *(See chapter four for specifics.)* Learning how to use your wheelchair, to transfer from chair to bed, and to perform your

---

SPINAL CORDS

CHOOSING A PERSONAL CARE ASSISTANT

Having someone help you with your daily routines can be liberating. It gives you more time to do the things you need and want to do. If you feel it's time to hire a personal care assistant, you're not alone. More than 40% of all SCI survivors have an assistant to help them do the laundry, cook their meals, straighten the house, and, if needed, to help with bathing, grooming, and brushing their teeth. Here are some hints when you're hiring:

- *Are you a "night owl" or a "lark?" If you don't have the finances to hire a full-time assistant, determine when you'll need help most. Maybe it's with your morning routines. Perhaps it's after work.*
- *Consolidate tasks so that you can "help yourself" later. Maybe she can make dinner and store it in the fridge for you. Maybe he can lay out your nightclothes for the evening before saying goodbye. Maybe she can put your clean clothes in the dryer, which you can easily pull out and put in a basket.*
- *Get advice from your rehabilitation team. They might be able to recommend someone. They'll point you toward funding resources, if necessary. They'll give you the facts you need for contracts and insurance. And, most importantly, they'll help you learn how to make your personal care assistant happy — so it will be a rewarding experience for the both of you.*

---

range-of-motion exercises can make all the difference in the way you relate — and function — in the world.

But there are a few functions that are "Still Required Reading" (SRR):

SRR #1: Feeding and Swallowing

Sometimes it's not just a matter of that cold glass of water just out of reach. It's not just being unable to use a knife and fork to cut some dark meat. If you have a C1 to C6 injury, it's possible that even if you could grab that glass or slice that turkey, you'd still not be able to swallow. High quad injuries can involve the neck and throat muscles; the nerves that signal the brain to send in saliva or start the mouth muscles chewing cannot get through. This condition is called dysphagia, and the good news is that we can do something about it. In addition to feeding tubes, your rehabilitation team will help you try to "retrain" those muscles. They might suggest sitting up when sipping through a tube or eating small bites of soft food that are easy to swallow. Electric stimulation can also help move those muscles.

SRR #2: Breathing

Chances are, if you have trouble swallowing, you may also have trouble breathing on your own. If your injury is in the high quad realm, you might need a ventilator in order to breathe. Your neck muscles, diaphragm, and abdominal muscles (which are also used for proper breathing) might not be working. If you have an injury from T1 to T12, it's possible that your chest muscles will not be able to help with the job. Your ability to breathe will be totally dependent on your neck and diaphragm.

Before 1940, an iron lung was the only option for those who couldn't breathe on their own; you'd be trapped in this tubelike apparatus from the neck down. Happily, today there are other options, including a plastic Pneumo-Wrap, a poncholike ventilator that you wear over your chest.

A better choice is a positive pressure ventilator. These are not only portable, battery operated, and less bulky, but they also help reduce the risk of respiratory infections. They are used in conjunction with tracheotomy, nasal, or mouth tubes.

Studies have found that many SCI survivors who initially need a ventilator may be able to breathe on their own several weeks or months after the injury. However, this is usually on a limited basis and precautions must be taken to avoid any respiratory problems. Some hints:

√ Get plenty of rest. If you are not using all your breathing power, you will get more easily fatigued — and more susceptible to infection.

√ Find a position that is the most comfortable for breathing. Although lung capacity is usually higher if you are sitting up, quadriplegics do better lying down.

√ A stomach corset can help your diaphragm move in and out.

√ Perform muscle-strengthening exercises. Your arms and legs are not the only parts of the body that need exercise. The muscles involved in breathing need to be made strong too. You'll not only breathe better, but you'll be able to fight fatigue more efficiently.

√ Medications, such as bronchodilators, can help keep the airways open. They have been found to improve lung function in survivors with cervical injuries.

√ Coughing. Clearing the lungs of mucous and other secretions keeps airway passages clear; it helps prevent such respiratory ailments as pneumonia and bronchitis. Without coughing regularly, you won't be able to clear your throat and lungs of secretions; congestion builds and respiratory failure can result. If you cannot cough on your own, have someone assist you. Lie down and have your caregiver push in on your stomach to get a cough going. "Clapping" the stomach with cuplike motions helps strengthen the chest cavity as well as get mucous up and out. FES therapy has also been found to induce a cough.

√ Stay trim and lean! Obesity makes breathing difficult in anyone, SCI survivors and the able-bodied alike. Keeping your body in shape with healthy foods and range-of-motion exercises will not only help you breathe but will take away the strain on your heart.

SRR #3: Dealing with Upper-Body Pain

Pain is no stranger to SCI survivors. Studies have found that up to 80% of those injured experience pain. And 41% claim that the pain is so severe that it interferes with their daily routines.

Aching arms, shoulders, and chests are by-products for many paraplegics. We call this the "overuse syndrome," which develops, well, from overuse. Pushing your wheelchair. Pulling yourself off the bed. Banging the keys on your keyboard. All these activities can cause strain in those muscles and joints you are constantly using.

You can't stop using those muscles nor would you want do. But you can take better care of yourself to avoid the pain of conditions such as: joint dysfunction, which can create immobility; posture problems, which can put added strain on the areas of your back that function; and thoracic outlet syndrome, which causes the muscles of your shoulder to tighten and painfully bear down on the nerves leading all the way down your arm. Carpal tunnel syndrome causes nerve pressure at the wrist and numbness in your hands. Other painful muscular and nervous conditions? Tennis elbow and bursitis.

How do you avoid pain? Think break — and not the kind that deals with bones. If you're at the computer, take time out to stretch every hour. If you've

---

SPINAL CORDS

A DOLL FOR THE MILLENNIUM

Barbie may have had her dream house, but the new American Girl of Today doll has her very own wheelchair. So does Barbie's friend Share a Smile Becky, which sold out within two weeks of hitting the shelves.

Today, more and more toy manufacturers are realizing that there is a market out there for children who are differently abled — and that includes kids with SCI. In fact, there are 20% more American children with some form of disability today than there were 10 years ago.

And things are only getting better. Apparently Barbie's dream house doesn't have the right dimensions to fit a wheelchair. Mattel received so many complaints that the dream house has been modified — and Becky is a frequent guest.

been pushing your wheelchair, stop for a moment and reflect. You might also consider switching to a power wheelchair if upper-body pain becomes too unmanageable.

And don't forget to exercise. Now, more than ever, you have to get in those stretches, especially those that emphasize the shoulder and the chest, range-of-motion exercises, proning, and resistance-training pulls and twists every day. Not only will exercise keep muscles supple and toned, joints strong and firm, but it will help ease strain — on your shoulders, arms, and back. You'll find yourself starting to sit up taller without even thinking about it.

REHABILITATION ENGINEERING

The words themselves might sound daunting, but rehabilitation engineering is something that should be close to your heart. It is, quite simply, a way to a better quality of life at home. A rehabilitation engineer helps design your home and workplace to conform to your needs. Ramps, grab bars, bathroom fixtures, door widths, entryways, work stations — these are all part of a day's work for the rehabilitation engineer. He will also help you with special wheelchair fittings. She will design and alter special seating. He will provide environmental controls, such as special light switches, heat and air controls, and alarm systems, to help you maintain independence in your house. (The majority of the time, your therapists can supply this information.)

Things that went unnoticed before your injury are now under scrutiny. How do you get into your house? How do you get up the stairs? How do you open the kitchen cupboards? The medicine chest? How do you go from room to room? How to get out fast in case of fire? How can you answer a ringing phone?

A room needs to be big enough for you to turn around in while sitting in your wheelchair. You need a sink that comes to your waist — not your neck. You need a doorway that is at least 30 inches wide to fit your wheelchair. You need a door with a latch that easily opens with one motion, as well as a kick plate on the bottom to protect the wood when it hits your footrest.

Your rehabilitation engineer will also make sure that your home and workspace are safe. Some hints:

- Keep ramps no steeper than 1 foot of length for each inch of height.
- Add protective shields or insulation to any exposed pipes and motors. You don't want to be surprised by a burn or scrape!
- Make sure you have at least two emergency exits in your home or office.
- Think outdoors for doors. They should never swing in as they can hit you and cause damage.
- Keep an alarm system nearby, a keypad, if possible, that links you to the fire department or police station with a button.

Although we've given you some solid information in this chapter, the main theme isn't miscellaneous at all. It's a matter that goes to the core of rehabilitation: independence. All the equipment, exercises, and suggestions we've introduced are designed for your independence, to help you function in the real world with all your potential intact.

But independence is not just a goal for you. It's something your loved one and caregiver must have as well in order to give you the help you need.

Let's go over their needs now.

SPINAL CORDS

A UNIVERSAL MESSAGE

"Optimism and humor are the grease and glue of life. Without both of them we would never have survived our captivity."

– Philip Butler, Vietnam POW

HELPING YOUR LOVED ONE MEANS HELPING YOURSELF: CAREGIVER RELIEF

"If you don't know how to help yourself, how can you know how to help anyone else?"

— Anonymous

"Okay, I admit it. Sometimes I hate my husband and his spinal cord injury. I am so tired of taking care of him!"

"There are so many things I have to do, from bathing and grooming to feeding, that there's no time left in the day for me!"

"When I close my eyes, I dream of freedom. No one to care for, no one to help. Just me."

"I'm losing patience with my wife. I know she's depressed because of her spinal cord injury. I know she can't help being in a wheelchair. But I get angry — and then comes the guilt. A vicious cycle."

"Call me selfish, but I need some space! Is there anyone out there who can help me?"

These are not the words of tyrants or evil villains. They are the voices of regular people, ordinary people like you and me, who happened to receive a terrible blow: The person they loved, their soul mate, husband, wife, or friend, had an accident which left them with a spinal cord injury. Even worse is the blame. Rehabilitation teams have heard over and over again mothers tearfully exclaim, "I wasn't even there." They weren't there to protect and comfort their child — in some cases, their adult children with families of their own. They believe, however irrational it is, that they could have done something.

Suddenly, their world and their place in it has turned upside-down. It's as if the accident had happened to them.

But it didn't. And, somehow, someway, these ordinary people, these heroes of everyday life, must find the strength, the energy, and the courage to help their loved one not only get through the rough spots, but the day-to-day routines.

SPINAL CORDS

SCI MYTH #8: GET USED TO YOUR NEW LIFE. YOU WON'T SEE ANY IMPROVEMENT IN YOUR LOVED ONE EVER

Reality is reality, and it is true that you have to eventually accept the fact that your loved one will not be the same again — ever. Depending on where the spinal cord injury occurred, he may never walk or control his bladder in the same way again.

But all is not grim. In fact, right after an SCI, the spinal cord is swollen and bruised, causing havoc throughout the body. But, eventually, within days or weeks, the swelling goes down, and it is possible that your loved one will regain some function.

Studies have also found that incomplete injuries have the best chance for improvement. Some functioning has returned to SCI survivors with incomplete injuries as much as a year and a half after the accident.

Remember that hope is motivating and strong. But false hope is ultimately debilitating. The best — and most promising — improvement comes from successful rehabilitation, one that helps your loved one develop the new skills for a new life.

Are you looking? Do you see them? Probably not. Most of us are understandably focused on the person with the spinal cord injury. But these people need help too.

This chapter is devoted to you, the caregiver, who is also in pain, to help you find and maintain the compassion, love, and resilience you need to do your best for your loved one.

A DIFFERENT SCENARIO

Susan had always considered herself a caring person. She was always ready to help her coworkers at the bank; she helped her mother with her chores. She volunteered for almost every committee at her son's school.

As busy as Susan was, her husband, Dave, was even busier. He not only shared the household chores with his wife, but he, too, worked full-time as an account executive at a local advertising agency. They took family vacations together; he coached his son's Little League team.

But as filled as Susan and Dave's life was, they always managed to grab a few hours here and there for a quiet dinner out or for a movie.

All in all, Susan felt blessed with her life — until it all fell apart with one wrong turn on a dark street. Dave had been coming home late from work; he'd been working on a presentation that was due the next day. He didn't see the car whose intoxicated driver neglected to see the stop sign on the corner.

The cars collided; Dave ended up with a C5-6 spinal cord injury. He needed to learn new skills for getting around, for his activities of daily living, for functional independence.

After six months of rehabilitation, the injury was behind him. He had made progress in using his wheelchair; he had his bladder and bowel program down to an efficient routine; he had become a whiz at the computer.

Susan had been there rooting for him the entire time Dave had been in the hospital. She'd given him the hope and inspiration he'd needed to get through the rough emotional waters. She, too, had gone into therapy to learn how to cope with her new life, to help her plan a new life for her family.

Susan knew that she'd have to curtail some of her volunteer work. Although they could afford a part-time personal care assistant, she still had to take care of grocery shopping, the laundry; she had to add an hour to any scheduled engagements to help Dave get dressed, to help him maneuver.

Then there was the budget to consider. Although Dave was doing well as a consultant working at home via his computer, he wasn't making as much as he had at the office. To cut corners, Susan quit her therapy. She also wanted to spend more quality time with their son; he'd begun acting out at school when his father had come home.

Things started to pile up. First it was only dirty clothes and dishes. But the more the school called Susan about her son, the more Dave asked her to come upstairs and help him, the more bills the postman dropped off, resentment, anger, and depression were added to the pile.

Susan was becoming overwhelmed. She began to scream at her son — and her husband. She'd run out to the car and roar out of the driveway without telling anyone where she was going.

She never went far. Susan would end up at a mall, an office parking lot, or a street nearby. She'd sit, her head on the steering wheel, and cry. And cry. Her sobs would fog up the windows. The guilt, the resentment, and the anger were almost palpable. Her once perfect life had turned into a nightmare.

STRESS, STRESS, AND MORE STRESS

Susan's uncontrollable spiral down to overwhelming despair didn't come out of the blue. Although you might be eternally grateful that your loved one is alive, you, too, probably have had all-too-human feelings of resentment, anger, and their accompanying guilt as the pressures mount.

Think about it. Your world, too, has changed dramatically. Your relation-

SPINAL CORDS

"The way I look at it, before I was paralyzed, there were ten thousand things I could do; ten thousand things I was capable of doing. Now, there are nine thousand. I can dwell on the one thousand, or concentrate on the nine thousand I have left. And, of course, the joke is that none of us in our lifetime is going to do more than two or three thousand of these things in any event."

– W. Mitchell, as quoted in
Options: Spinal Cord Injury and the Future
by Barry Corbet
Denver: Hirschfeld Press, 1980.

ship with your loved one has changed — physically and mentally. Your personal time and space has gotten smaller as a direct result of the spinal cord damage done. Your friends and family might all have good intentions, but they can't completely understand how it feels to have your sex life, your bathroom routines, your personal time so completely different — and out of your control. Then there is the endless worry, the financial fears, the burden of responsibility, the anxiety that your loved one might develop an infection, a pressure sore, or autonomic dysreflexia.

Social isolation. Continuous anxiety. A lack of boundaries. Traumatic change. All these contribute to an unbearable feeling of psychic pain. Out of control and out of your element, you might find yourself sinking into a terrible depression — where no one gets better.

Although these feelings make sense, they don't have to be engraved in your heart. They are not etched in stone.

It doesn't have to be this way.

HOPE: FUEL FOR THE SOUL

Fortunately, Susan's story has a happy ending. She finally realized that she couldn't handle the stress on her own. She joined a support group which helped her find new resources: an outpatient clinic, discount supplies, and a wide network of new friends. Susan was no longer alone. She had people around her who understood. Her stress levels relieved, Susan was able to handle her responsibilities at home. Everybody benefited.

Although Susan's story is not an unusual one, not every story ends on an uplifting note. Many caregivers do not get the help they need. They become more and more depressed until they flee or get mired down in a life of despair, all the while the person with spinal cord injury they'd once loved feels trapped, angry, hopeless, and resentful as well.

Your situation doesn't have to have the sad ending. You can be an excellent caregiver — without giving up your life. You can be loving and compassionate — and selfish. Everyone can wind up happy. Here are some suggestions, some "caregiver credos" that have helped many of our family members:

Caregiver Credo #1: Time Out!

The phone doesn't ring when it's convenient for you. Your job doesn't start when you feel like coming into the office. You don't get a cold or the flu when you could use a few days off. Never! Life's routines, its ups and downs, its comings and goings, are not governed by you — unless you grab some control for yourself.

Making time for yourself is a way of gaining that control, which is especially important if you are a caregiver. When you are administering to someone else's needs, it's easy to forget yours. Time has a way of slipping through your fingers as you make dinner, transfer your husband or wife from wheelchair to bed, as you deal with all the other daily odds and ends.

Arrange for a personal care assistant to come over for a few hours in the morning or afternoon, whichever time is best for *you*. Use this free time selfishly and completely for yourself. Put the answering machine on and turn off the phone's ringer. Take a bath or use this quiet time reading or taking a nap. Learn how to meditate. If it's a beautiful day and the house is feeling cramped, get out! Go for a walk or a massage. Get your hair done. Take a class in a subject you've always wanted to learn: watercolor, pottery, or even 18th-century English lit! Whatever. The important message in this credo is the medium: you. It's your time out to refuel, replenish, and regroup.

Caregiver Credo #2: A Physical Labor of Love

It's not just the SCI survivor who needs to exercise and eat right. You do too. More and more people are beginning to realize that it's not enough to study hard and work the brain. Your body needs muscle too. A sound body will help calm your mind. Exercise not only helps relieve some of the frustration and stress you feel, it also makes you stronger — and better able to handle the physical aspects of your caregiving role.

Eating a well-balanced, nutritious diet will also help keep your strength up and your stress levels down. Sugar makes you jittery — a quick surge and an equally quick slump. Better to eat complex carbohydrates, such as whole grain breads, sweet potatoes, and rice; protein; and plenty of sweet fruits and vegetables. You'll get the vitamins, minerals, and fiber you need — without the "sugar drop." Suddenly, you'll also find that you are able to make that bed with gusto, tell a funny joke and really laugh, and help with range-of-motion exercises with a lot more energy than you ever thought you had!

Caregiver Credo #3: Education is Power

In the very beginning of this book, we talked about the strength found in knowledge. If you've learned nothing else from these pages, we hope you'll have taken away the need for information, for education. SCI survivors need this knowledge in order to facilitate the rehabilitation process. The more they know, the better it will work — and the more motivated they will stay.

The same goes for you. Take advantage of your loved one's rehabilitation center. Ask your case manager and others on the rehabilitation team any questions you might have. Don't be embarrassed; they've most likely heard it all before!

Join a spinal cord injury network, such as the National Spinal Cord Injury Association. They can give you good, sound advice on everything from personal care assistants to financial aid. (You'll find their address, phone numbers, and Web site in appendix C at the back of this book.)

Read this book — and others. Learn as much as you can. The more you know, the better you'll understand and the stronger you will feel.

Caregiver Credo #4: Therapy

A good counselor to help you discover coping strategies is vital for your well-being, and, ultimately, the well-being of your loved one. Your rehabilitation hospital can help you find someone who specializes in spinal cord injury survivors and their caregivers. In fact, a good rehabilitation hospital will have a counselor on staff as part of the team. (See chapter three on rehabilitation.)

Support groups are also part of that therapeutic process. You are not only among people who understand what you are going through — they are going through it themselves! Support groups can help relieve your isolation. They

---

SPINAL CORDS

BE THE HOST WITH THE MOST

The last thing you might feel like doing is playing host to your friends or family. But a party might be just what you need. Studies have found that caregivers who get lots of visitors have less stress than those who never hear the doorbell ring.

Entertaining doesn't have to impress Martha Stewart. You can make sandwiches or serve iced tea, cold vegetables, and chips. Better yet, have your guests bring a dish that everyone can share. An added plus: Your loved one will enjoy the company too.

can act as a "pressure cooker valve," giving you a chance to vent your feelings.

Even more important: A support group made up of your peers will be a valuable resource for you, a place to share and find out information. You'll be able to find out firsthand if a particular personal care assistant is good, if a certain van is the best buy for the money, or if the contractor you found to add disabled-accessible features to your home is reliable.

These are only a few "caregiver credos," but they all come down to one thing: Are you taking care of yourself? Take a moment and think about it. Use your common sense — and your instincts. What do you want to do? How can you fit it into your life? Remember, if you aren't making yourself happy, you won't be any good to anyone else. No one likes a martyr — especially the SCI survivor who loves you.

Our journey together is almost over. But before we close, we'd like to take a few questions — and answers.

C H A P T E R   T W E L V E

HELP! QUESTIONS AND ANSWERS TO COMMON PROBLEMS AND SITUATIONS

"The more questions I ask, the more I learn. The more I learn, the stronger I feel. And, at least for me, there's no better feeling in the world."

— An 18-year-old SCI survivor who
had an L2 injury while rock climbing

It's a paradox: The more you learn, the more you need to know. Questions help you understand the complexities you couldn't grasp in the beginning. They help put what you learned into perspective, to make general themes specific to you and your situation. To help you assimilate the information you gathered in this book, to help what you learned become part of your everyday life, here are some of the common questions we've heard time and again as we've helped spinal cord injury survivors and their families adjust to their new lives.

▶ *How do I know when I have a urinary tract infection — and how can I keep them from recurring?*
If you have a urinary tract infection (UTI), you are not alone. Studies have found that the most common medical complication following a spinal cord injury is UTI. Approximately 80% of all SCI survivors suffer from a UTI at one time or another within a year after their injury. Symptoms include:
- Cloudy or smelly urine
- Fever
- Sweating and chills
- Blood in the urine
- More voiding than normal in your usual bladder management program
- Leaking around your catheter
- A burning feeling when voiding

Although urinary tract infections are common in the able-bodied as well, they can become more serious in people with SCI. Since you cannot tell when your bladder is full, you might not be able to recognize the symptoms until they are more serious, possibly leading to kidney disease.

The best treatment is prevention. Make sure you clean your equipment after each use. Wash your hands before and after voiding. Check your catheter frequently to make sure it is working properly. Make sure you empty your bladder fully every time you void. A too-full bladder can make you vulnerable to infection.

Caregiver Tip: Make sure your loved one is keeping to his bladder management routine. Check that she is keeping her catheter clean. If you feel there is any reason to suspect a UTI, don't hesitate to act. Bring a urine sample to your physician.

▶ *How can I control spasms in my legs? They jerk and tighten up at the most inconvenient times. It's embarrassing!*

Another common complication of spinal cord injury is spasticity. These muscle spasms are, literally, exaggerated muscle tension, a result of your damaged spinal cord. Messages to your nerves and muscles are not properly transmitted. Your legs or arms are not only paralyzed, unable to move, but they can also move (jerk or tighten) out of the blue. Spasticity can occur in just about anyone who has had a spinal cord injury.

Some spasticity is even welcome. It helps tone muscles and keeps them strong. If your jerks are not too frequent and uncomfortable, your physician might not even prescribe medication to keep them at bay.

However, if your spasticity is getting in the way of your independence, antispasmodic medication, such as dantrolene (Dantrium), baclofen (Lioresal), or tizanidine (Zanaflex), can be prescribed. In severe cases, baclofen is administered automatically into the spinal fluid via an injection pump that is inserted near your stomach, just below your skin. This not only prevents spasms, but it also helps control some of the side effects of baclofen, such as nausea, vomiting, and fatigue.

Caregiver Tip: Medication is not the only route to take. A change of posture can also help control spasms. Studies have found that a standing position can help reduce spasticity. Help your loved one move; make sure he does his range-of-motion exercises and his stretches. He might be able to control his spasticity with less medication.

▶ *Can I still have children?*

The good news is that there may be no reason why you can't have children if you have a spinal cord injury. Although sexual function might be affected by your injury, adjustments and techniques can be made to help ensure a healthy sex life. However, SCI can cause some complications. Studies have found that men may produce less sperm and those they do ejaculate may not be as "energetic." However, harvesting sperm through vibratory stimulation or a process called electroejaculation (which, in turn, can be used for artificial insemination and in vitro fertilization) can help prevent male infertility. Retroejaculation is a similar process; the sperm is harvested via the bladder.

Most women have no problems with fertility, even though menstruation may stop for a few months from the physical trauma of SCI. Their problems occur during pregnancy. If you get pregnant, it's important that your physician supervises you closely to avoid urinary tract infections, anemia, premature birth, and autonomic dysreflexia — which is not only dangerous in its own right, but because it has been confused with labor.

Caregiver Tip: Women with SCI above T10 do not always know they are going into labor. Watch carefully for the signs as the date approaches. Shortness of breath, muscle spasms, and back pain can all be symptoms of labor, which is usually shorter in woman with SCI.

▶ *How can I meet new people? How can I find someone to date who won't pity me — or worse?*

You don't have to have a spinal cord injury to feel isolated and alone. Many able-bodied spend more than one Saturday night eating a frozen dinner in front of the tube instead of dancing the night away at the newest club.

Like able-bodied people, it might not be easy to meet someone if you have SCI. And, yes, part of it is the injury itself. Unfortunately, many people still think of SCI survivors in wheelchairs as invalids and victims of tragic accidents. Until we change the language we use and the prejudices that give it voice, there will always be those who pity you or act condescendingly.

But, for every person who doesn't understand, there are many who do; interesting, vital people who share your interests and want to meet you. One of the best places to meet new friends is through a support group. Ask your rehabilitation hospital if they know of any in the area. Check out your local cable station, the ads in your local paper, and your local church. And don't forget the convenience of the Web.

If there isn't a group in your area, start your own! Contact your rehabilitation center. Ask them to contact other survivors. They might even send out mailers for you — and pay for the postage. Your local church or community center may donate space for your group's meetings.

Caregiver Tip: Be sensitive to your loved one's moods. If he seems very lonely, spiraling into feelings of hopelessness, you should contact the rehabilitation center. He might need to see a therapist more frequently or take some medication.

▶ *Before my accident, I was in construction. I need a new job with different skills. Any suggestions?*

When it comes to work, some SCI survivors are more fortunate than others. If you had a "desk job" before your accident, chances are your office can be accommodated to meet your new needs. In fact, your workplace, if in a new building, must be disabled-accessible by law: The Americans with Disabilities Act (ADA). (Unfortunately, if a building is older, the owners may not have to comply; they can claim the changes are too "unreasonable" and financially taxing.)

If your work was more physical, requiring you to climb or move around in ways that are just not practical with a wheelchair, you will have to rethink what you want to do. Rather than thinking you have to "start over," that it's hopeless and overwhelming, be positive. Think of your new career as a new opportunity. You might even like it better than your old work life!

To help you determine "where to go from here," you might want to talk to your vocational counselor and your occupational therapist at the rehabilitation center. They are trained to help you learn new skills, to train for a new job. You'll learn how to gear your abilities and interests to a specific job. And you'll also learn more effective ways to find that new job.

There are also state and national Job Training Programs (JTP) that may help out financially. The national Office of Vocational Rehabilitation (OVR) may also help. They may pay to send you to school to learn a new job — a great plus for someone who is considering you for a job! Ask your vocational therapist about training programs in your area.

Caregiver Tip: Encourage your loved one to try new things. If you have a computer, let her at it! There are some excellent software programs to learn typing, bookkeeping, and management. There are also devices, such as mouthpicks, book racks, turntable desks, and ratchet wrist-hand orthoses, to help with "desk jobs."

▶ *I've heard that people with SCI age faster than the able-bodied. How can I stop the process? How can I keep strong and healthy?*

The hard fact is that it's true: SCI survivors have to work harder at keeping complications, illness, and aging at bay. But things are getting better all the time. Before World War II, most people who had a spinal cord injury weren't expected to last longer than a few weeks. Urinary problems, pressure sores, and infection usually did them in. But today, with new antibiotics, state-of-the-art products and devices, and responsible, knowledgeable rehabilitation, SCI survivors can live a much longer and healthier life than in the past.

However, your situation does require more vigilance. In the same way you must perform your bladder and bowel management programs, your daily

---

SPINAL CORDS

BABY STEPS, BABY STEPS

If you are taking care of someone who's had an SCI and he seems to have lost all his confidence, don't lose hope. Think baby steps. If you can get him to take a bus by himself, drive a car to the store, ride the train to the next town, he'll feel great; his sense of accomplishment will follow through to other areas of his life.

Today, the car. Tomorrow, the community at large. The more she does by herself, the more she'll want to do. That first ride around the block in a new van can lead to getting a job or going back to school.

---

range-of-motion exercises, you must also watch for signs of complications due to your particular injury.

SCI survivors are more at risk for osteoporosis, a condition when bones become brittle and weak. The result can be fractures, broken bones, and pain. For SCI survivors, this can translate into a loss of function as well as an increased risk for skin and respiratory complications if you can no longer sit up.

Why osteoporosis? Almost immediately after your injury, your bones begin to lose vital minerals and become weak. This might be caused by the strong steroid medicine you are taking, diabetes, smoking, too much alcohol or caffeine, and, most crucial of all, inactivity. Perhaps you are not exercising your limbs; you are spending a lot of time in bed. Perhaps you are not performing weight-bearing exercises that help make bones strong. Further, studies have found that the changes in your circulatory and nervous system create chemical imbalances. After an injury, your body actually eliminates vital minerals from your bones. The proof is the mineral content found in excreted urine.

All is not bleak. The "mineral dump" usually stops after two years. Further, osteoporosis does not make broken bones a foregone conclusion. You don't have to have a fracture! In fact, only 6% of SCI survivors do.

To help stave off the effects of osteoporosis, make sure you do your exercises every day, especially weight-bearing routines with the help of another person — your therapist or a caregiver. Take a calcium and magnesium supplement under your doctor's supervision. (The magnesium helps the bones absorb the calcium.) Drink more milk and eat more broccoli. Both are loaded with calcium! Ditto for fish and green, leafy vegetables for vitamin D.

Caregiver Tip: Optimal health will keep your loved one strong and keep the aging process at a slow pace. Keep a watchful eye and make sure he goes in for checkups on a regular basis. Try to get her to stop smoking. Help him ease up on the alcohol. (But be diplomatic. Nagging doesn't work!)

Physical health is only part of the picture. Make sure your loved one is intellectually stimulated, that there are people around for him to talk to and love. Make sure she is emotionally stable, that she is taking her medicine, if necessary, and getting the help she needs to cope with her injury. And, above all, take care of yourself. Remember, you can't love anyone else if you don't love yourself!

▶ *I want to get a van, but where do I start? Will it really help with my driving?*

Let's face it. Being able to drive a car means freedom. Getting behind the wheel, pushing down on the pedal, driving along a country road with the wind in your hair all spell freedom and, especially for SCI survivors, movement. Car companies have long recognized their vehicles as symbols for freedom. Witness the number of ads showing these images!

But after a spinal cord injury, driving in your car might become cumbersome, inconvenient, and even hazardous to your health. One of the biggest complaints people with SCI have is shoulder pain and fatigue. These ailments are increased by transferring to the driver's side of the car, by getting in and out of the car, and by sitting in a seat that is too low or too short.

Vans can help reduce shoulder pain and fatigue and, by doing so, promote a healthier, happier frame of mind. Vans use lifts to simply and easily get you up and into the driver's seat. The steering wheel and seat are specifically designed to ease the tension in your wrists and arms; hand controls replace the brake and gas pedals. Once you've learned how to drive the bigger vehicle, you'll fit right in. Recreational vehicles (RVs) are hot!

One point: Vans do cost more money, both initially and for fuel. Minivans are hard to adapt, especially if the floor needs to be dropped and a lift is needed. A better choice is a conversion van. Not only is it easier to adapt for people with SCI, but the purchase of the vehicle and its modifications are tax-free. If you need help in financing your van, talk to your rehabilitation team about contacting car dealerships that might have a special program to help fund adaptations.

Caregiver Tip: Help your loved one choose a van that's also something you'll feel comfortable in. A van can spell freedom for you as well, making transfers and positioning much easier and more efficient.

▶ *Help! I'm gaining weight sitting in this wheelchair all day.*

Before we say anything else, let's dispel this popular myth: No, you don't have to gain weight if you have a spinal cord injury. One study of SCI survivors between the ages of 20 and 50 found that the majority of people only gained 1 pound a year! In fact, you will probably lose weight at first. Your body goes into shock; you aren't eating as much as you normally do; you are in an emergency situation.

But some people will gain weight — just as many able-bodied do as they age. The only problem is that along with the usual list of complaints — high blood pressure, high cholesterol, gall bladder disease, arthritis, and diabetes — people with SCI have an added roster: more pressure sores, less bladder control, constipation, more circulatory complications, fatigue, shoulder pain, and an even greater loss of self-esteem.

If you are obese, you also will be less able and willing to do your daily functions. You'll have to hire more full-time help to get you dressed, moving, and on your way. Even worse, you'll find it harder to find that help. Some personal care assistants cannot work with obese patients; it's very hard on their backs.

Although your metabolism does change after SCI and you expend less energy, you can win the battle of the bulge. And the "magic formula" is the same for you as it is for the able-bodied: diet and exercise. Eat a healthy, low-fat, high-fiber diet, chock-full of fruits and vegetables. Stay away from sugary, starchy desserts and alcohol. Try eating several small meals a day; it can help "trick" your metabolism into staying strong. And do the exercises you learned in physical therapy every day!

Caregiver Tip: A person has to want to lose weight for himself. You cannot "get" her to lose weight any more than you can "get" her to quit smoking. But you can provide a consistent, reliable, and inspirational presence. Cook meals that are low in fat but also delicious. (There are many books out today that offer fast, healthy meals.) Leave the desserts and the liquor on the store shelves. Exercise yourself! Everyone can use more movement in their lives.

▶ *I'm getting older. How do I know when I'm ready to give up my manual wheelchair for a power chair? Is it really a sign of giving up my independence?*

Many SCI survivors see their manual wheelchair as a sign of independence. Pushing on those wheels, moving those strong arm muscles, turning on your own — these all feel like independence, of self-control. Changing to a power chair, mechanical and easy, feels like giving up, of losing that important control and independence. And it's true that, in the beginning, rehabilitation patients are encouraged to use a manual chair. The pushing motion is initially very important to keep up activity levels, strength, and endurance. But laziness is one thing — and age is another. If you are young and vital, but want to use a power chair right from the start, you're letting your "couch potato" tendencies get in the way of your independence. But if you are older and using your manual chair is a struggle, a power chair can be the best option around. Don't be stubborn — and don't think of it as "giving up."

This negative way of thinking hurts you — and those you love. After many years of pushing a manual chair, those arm muscles take a beating. Maybe you have less upper-body strength than you used to have. Maybe you are very, very tired. Maybe you can't get around as easily as you once did, and you end up staying home a lot.

Yes, change is hard, but think about it. Aren't you losing more independence by staying home, by feeling bad, by needing more sleep, by being in pain? A power chair can actually mean independence!

Just ask 59% of the SCI survivors who participated in a study in England. They changed equipment and were able to maintain their same quality of functional independence, mobility, and sense of well-being. Even better: Their shoulder pain and fatigue decreased. How do you know if it's time to change? Here's a check list:

√ Do you avoid going places you used to love to visit?
√ Do you find yourself using up all your energy doing such simple activities as going from room to room?
√ Do you have less shoulder pain and feel less tired when you've been out of your wheelchair for a while?
√ Does your shoulder always hurt when you are in your wheelchair?

If you've answered yes to any of these questions, discuss the pros and cons of a power chair with your therapist.

Just as the able-bodied can no longer dance till dawn in their 50s, middle-aged SCI survivors can no longer move about as swiftly as they did in their teens.

Caregiver Tip: Remember, your needs are important too. Chances are that if your loved one no longer has the energy he had as a young man, you don't either. Maybe pushing and guiding that manual chair has become an exhausting task for you as well. Make your needs known. Tell your loved one how you feel. You should be part of the decision.

▶ *I used to love to travel. Do I have to give it up now that I have a spinal cord injury?*

Absolutely not! You might have to do a bit more planning ahead of time, but you can certainly enjoy visiting new places as much as you did before. Here are some hints to help you "pack light":

√ Find a good travel agency well in advance of your travel plans. Make sure they have experience with SCI survivors. These agencies will know in advance which hotels have appropriate door widths, ramps, and grab bars. Most hotels have disabled-accessible rooms. (And don't forget to make it a nonsmoking room too!)

√ Make a list of everything you'll need for your trip, including medical supplies and equipment. Buy baggage that will accommodate everything without weighing you down.

√ If you have a power wheelchair, make sure you bring along extra batteries!

√ Check for medical supply stores and wheelchair repair companies in the cities you'll be visiting — just in case.

√ Try to book direct flights on all airlines, if possible — unless you need to deplane to change your catheter.

√ Don't check your wheelchair until you get to the gate. This way you'll have your mobility right before you get on the plane.

√ Call your airline in advance to determine accessibility. You might have to bring a portable wheelchair.

√ A hint: Try not to drink your usual amount of water before air travel. A little dehydration will mean your bladder won't get too full at an inconvenient time. (But always check with your doctor before changing any routines! Dehydration can be dangerous if not closely monitored.)

√ Do your homework. Read about the cities or countryside you'll be visiting. Will there be a lot of cobblestone streets? They can play havoc with wheelchairs! What about puddles and muddy streets? Are most of the tourist sites wheelchair accessible?

√ Investigate travel resources for people with SCI, such as Flying Wheel at (800) 535-6790 or by fax at (507) 451-5005. Mobility International, which specializes in finding overseas jobs for people in wheelchairs, can be reached at (541) 343-6812 or by fax at (541) 343-1284. You can also reach Mobility International by e-mail at info@miusa.org or via their Web site: www.miusa.org. Check out travel Web sites for more information too.

These are only a few of the questions we get every day. You might have other concerns. Don't hesitate to ask your rehabilitation team anything that comes to mind. Remember: In knowledge, there is strength. And with strength comes independence.

THE STRENGTH OF THE SPIRIT CAN PREVAIL

Jimmy wanted to fly.

Susan wanted to run down the hall, her hands in the air.

Sam wanted to go back in time, before his accident.

June simply wanted to breathe, in and out, without thinking about it.

Everyone who has had a spinal cord injury has their dream, their wish, and it always comes down to one thing: to be like before, to walk, to feel, and to be as you were before the accident. It's replayed over and over again. "Why did I...How come I...If only I had...."

But, eventually, reality takes hold. Common sense tells you that life cannot be the way it was. Life is full of surprising twists of fate, of events that change everything within seconds. You had a spinal cord injury. Yes. You cannot go backward.

But it is not the end.

Rather, it is another beginning, a new place where you can learn new ways to be, to maneuver, to be independent.

Life does not have to stop with spinal cord injury. If there's one thing we wanted to show you in this book, it is this: Life is not over. You can get back.

Reality changes every day. Snow turns to rain. Snow melts. People age. There is also the miracle of a new day, of feeling the sun on your face — of being alive. You have that opportunity, that feeling. You can still greet a new day. Your mind is hearty and strong. You can conquer anything, including despair. Hold on, and get back to a healthy, normal, functional life. It is within your grasp.

Within these pages, we've shown you the basics of spinal cord injury. We've taken you from the injury itself through the many arenas involved in rehabilitation and beyond. We hope you have learned something. We also hope you've learned that you can reclaim hope: You can leave the despair you may now feel and find determination and optimism waiting inside, ready to be heard.

You didn't plan your spinal cord injury. You can't control the accidents that occur. But you can control the way you handle it. You can control your life.

To that life. And all the possibilities it still holds.

We wish you well.

WHEN YOU LEAVE REHABILITATION: EQUIPMENT YOU MAY NEED FOR LIVING

For your bed
Loop chains or bed ladders
Leg loops
A hospital bed
Special pressure reduction mattress

For transfers
Sliding board
Leg loops

For your home
Ramps for two good exits (1-foot incline per every 1 inch in height)
Wider doorways
Rearranged furniture and rugs for easy access
Special door handles
Accessible door locks
Accessible phone
Accessible appliance controls

For your bathroom
Grab bars near the toilet, tub, and shower
Roll-in shower
Roll-in shower chair
Cabinet cutouts
Pocket door
Faucet and door handles
Hand-held shower with adaptive handle
Soap dispenser in tub and shower
Tub bench

Adaptive bathing and catheter equipment
Flip-top squeeze toothpaste and adaptive toothbrush
Adaptive hairbrush

For your wheelchair
Rigid frame or sturdy lightweight frame
Power wheelchair with tilt and recline ability
Drive controls for power wheelchair
Cushion offering best position and pressure relief
Push gloves for manual wheelchair

For your car
Drive controls adapted to your style and effort. Zero gravity, if necessary.
Handicap parking placard and/or license plate
A van or modified car
Van lift
Six-way seat for van
Lock down for van
Device to lower floor and raise roof
License with restriction change. Driving school attendance, if necessary
Public transportation permit, if necessary

For exercise
A standing frame
Helm® gym or Versatrainer®, a wheelchair-accessible weight system
Wheelchair roller
Weights
Pulleys
Thera-Band® elastic exercise bands
ERGYS® system or StimMaster Ergometer® for Functional Electrical Stimulation (FES)
Respond, an electrical stimulation unit
Powder board and skate
Mat

APPENDIX B

WHAT TO LOOK FOR IN A WHEELCHAIR

Work with your therapist to determine your specific needs. Areas to consider include:

Personal Requirements

Weight: If you are heavy, you may need a wider chair with durable pneumatic tires and a reinforced frame.

Spasticity Relief: If severely spastic, you'll need a chair with more trunk and limb support and more safety features.

Pressure Sore Relief: Depending on manual ability, you may need either a power recline and tilt system or simple assistive straps bolted to the chair.

Manual Independence: A manual chair usually works for all people with SCI, even if quadriplegic. However, a power chair may be necessary for long distances and for some quadriplegia conditions.

Health: If you have a pressure ulcer, you need to have a modified seat. If you have arthritis or heart disease, you might not be able to handle a manual chair. If you have had a head injury, you might not be able to use complicated, high-tech chairs. If your body remains rigid, in a straight position (orthostatic), you will need a recliner and possibly elevated legrests. If you have no head control, you'll need a recliner or Tilt-in-Space chair with headrest.

Propulsion: Your chair will need to be adjusted to the way you move, either with one leg, one leg and one arm, both legs, one arm, or both arms. Limbs that do not function need to be supported.

Strength and Endurance: Conventional wheelchairs weigh 40 to 50 pounds. Lightweight chairs weigh between 20 and 29 pounds. Which will be easier for you to manage?

Daily Environment: The terrain you travel is critical. If you frequently move on rocky or unpaved streets, your wheelchair must be durable. If you are indoors more often than not, your parts do not have to be as strong. If you are in your chair all day, it must be comfortable. And you must be able to relieve pressure! If you travel long distances, you might consider a power chair. Ditto for getting quickly to your job or from class to class.

Financial Concerns: If you cannot afford the wheelchair that is best for you, don't settle for just any model. There may be state or charitable funding. The vendor might agree to a payment plan. Speak to your case manager about options.

TYPES OF WHEELCHAIRS

Lightweights. For people with minimum spasticity and average seating capability. Some specifics:

- *Weight:* Approximately 20-30 pounds.
- *Folding:* Crossbars under seat allow chair to fold lengthwise. Less stable than rigid chair.
- *Rigid Chair:* Still has quick-release wheels and a fold-forward back for placing in car. More durable than folding chair.
- *Frame Composition:* Aluminum alloy, stainless steel, titanium (carbon fiber) — the lightest and most expensive — and now, the newest, no-tools necessary wheelchair, the Quickie TNT.
- *Frame Length:* The shorter the length, the more maneuverable the chair, allowing for more ease in getting close to doors, tables, desks, and counters. Length should be at an 80-degree angle, allowing knees to be at 90 degrees.
- *Chair Height from Floor:* Most chairs are "hemi-height" or "low-rider." Best for people who can propel chairs with at least one leg or for amputees who need to have prosthesis touch the ground when sitting. Height range should be 19 inches to 21 inches from floor to seat rail.
- *Sling Seat Depth and Width:* Vary in width from 14 inches to 20 inches. Depth determined by leg length from knee to hip. Can be customized for additional cost.
- *Backrests:* Recliner or rigid chairs usually adjustable from angle of 0 degrees to 8 degrees. Although not particularly helpful for balance, the 8 degrees can provide a greater degree of functional independence for people who need it. Rigid chairs also have backrests that fold forward. Can come with "quad" release mechanisms to facilitate folding.
- *Upholstery:* Either vinyl, nylon, Naugahyde, or "parapack" — a type of nylon that stretches the least.
- *Axles:* Quick release, with a push button mechanism located at hub of wheel to remove wheel from axle; quad release, for people with poor hand function; or threaded axle, which uses a long bolt to attach wheel to axle

and can only be removed with tools. Can be adjusted for amputees by ordering an "amputee frame" where the axle plate is extended in the rear.

- *Wheels:* There are two types. *Spoked wheels,* like a bicycle, are easy to use and very light, but require frequent "strumming" or tuning to make sure wheels are not warped. Radial spokes branch out from a center in a ray-like formation. Regular spokes cross over each other as they radiate out. *"Mag" (magnesium) polycarbon plastic molded rays* are heavier, but only need to be cleaned. If a spoked wheel gets bent, only the damaged spokes need to be replaced. If a "mag" wheel gets bent, the entire wheel must be replaced.

- *Tires:* There are five types. Pneumatic tires are just like bicycle tires, complete with inner air tube prone to punctures and flats. Good for all terrain and very light. Semipneumatics are very similar, but their inner tubes contain preformed polyurethane fillers, called foam inserts, which make them more durable. Good for all terrain and very light. Hard rubber tires are heavier. Encapsulated rubber tires have air space at center of rubber. Tubular latex tires are also known as "turbo tires," "continentals," or "court tires." Made of a different type of rubber than the other tires, these have no inner tube; they can still hold air at high pressures. Good for fast movement on smooth surfaces.

- *Handrims:* Either made of aluminum or stainless steel. Most lightweights are made with aluminum. Plastic-coated handrims are good for people with poor handgrip; they increase friction during a stroke. Also good in the rain. Handrim projections or "quad pegs" are cumbersome, but help if handgrip is very poor. Good for rough carpets or moving down a ramp.

- *Wheel Locks (Brakes):* Toggles need a push or pull to lock. Scissor brakes consist of crisscrossed levers. High-mount scissor brakes are the most flexible. They allow fast and full movement without having to move too far forward. Low-mount brakes keep fingers away from locks. Any scissor brake is good for transfers.You can now get a toggle that pushes forward to a horizontal position, keeping it out of the way. Spring-loaded brakes offer a stronger hold. Push/pull brakes have between 6-inch and 9-inch removable extensions that help people with muscle tone or balance problems. Unilateral extensions enable people with same arm and same leg paralysis (hemiplegics) to reach across with their functional arm to the opposite break.

- *Casters:* The two small wheels at the front of wheelchair. Diameter ranges from 3 inches to 6 inches. The wider the diameter, the rougher the ride. Eight-inch casters are rarely ordered, even if you won't be using the wheelchair very often. They get in the way when you are turning and they tend to "dip" their heels. Casters are made of hard polyurethane plastic, best for smooth surfaces, or the same materials used in tires: hard rubber, pneumatic and semipneumatic. The pneumatics are more comfortable on rough terrain. The newest casters are tiny plastic ones, similar to those on in-line skates, which don't require any maintenance.

- *Armrests:* These can be either slip-on tubes or slots along sides of chair. Can also consist of tubes that are only attached at the back, "standing free" in front. Slots come full-length, partial, or desk length. Tubes are only available in desk length; they are not too long. Both can be height adjustable. Lever systems, drop slots, swing away mechanisms, and pivots can be used to customize the chair and height.
- *Front Riggings:* These are the legrests, either fixed with one rigid footplate or fixed with flip-up footplate. Plates are length adjustable. Legrests may swing away. Main factors in choosing: ability to transfer and to manage legs. Also consider which front rigging allows for a 90-degree knee bend when you sit. Do you sit and stand frequently? A rigid footplate is usually not in the way for either sitting or standing.

Conventional Wheelchairs. Weighs 50 pounds if made of chrome-plated steel or 40 pounds if made of stainless steel. Fewer choices than lightweight. These are only good in institutions or if you cannot afford a lightweight chair. Even if someone pushes it, lightweight is best. Only available accessories are seat belts and anti-tip tubes. This is *not* a custom wheelchair! Some specifics:

- *Push Handles:* Always present.
- *Backrest:* Fixed at 16 to 17 inches in height. Can have manual reclining feature with removable headrest. This feature is best used in the rehabilitation hospital. Caution must be used as chair can tip when in a horizontal position or if you are doing a lot of steering.
- *Upholstery:* Vinyl or Naugahyde.
- *Armrests:* May be fixed or removable. May be adjustable in height. Can come in full or desk length. Includes metal or plastic panel to protect clothes from dirty tires.
- *Legrests:* May be elevated, swing away, or fixed with flip-up footplates.
- *Footrests:* Adjustable in length and rotation.
- *Wheel Locks:* High-mounted toggles.
- *Hand Rims:* Chrome-plated steel.
- *Tires:* Pneumatic or hard rubber.

Power Wheelchairs. Best for people with limited physical ability but intact cognitive ability. There are four types:

- *Belt-Driven:* Belt connects motor to wheel. Motor turns belt and the belt turns the wheel, providing rear wheel drive. Affords ample space under seat for easy accommodation of life-support equipment.
- *Direct Drive:* No belts. Motor directly turns wheel; either front or rear wheel

drive. Front wheel drive is best over rough terrain. More powerful than belt-driven and can also accommodate life-support equipment.

- *Power Base:* Also direct drive and most powerful of all. Look like small tractors with four wide pneumatic tires. Made for active people in the great outdoors

- *Friction Drive:* Also called "add-on system." Power component is added on to manual chair. Motor turns a set of rollers. Rollers contact the wheels and turn them. Most portable and least expensive. Another advantage: If power drive breaks down, the manual chair is a "back-up." Disadvantages: Noisy, less powerful, frequent replacement of tires necessary, rollers become slippery and dangerous when wet, and possible warranty limitations. Only works well on conventional wheelchairs. Too heavy for lightweight chairs (makes them "tip").

(See chapter five on mobility for more information on power wheelchair accessories such as headswitches, joysticks, and puff sticks.)

A P P E N D I X   C

COMMUNITY AND NATIONAL RESOURCES FOR HELP

American Association of People with Disabilities
1819 H Street, N.W.
Suite 330
Washington, DC 20006
(800) 840-8844
(202) 457-8168
(202) 457-0473 (fax)
www.aapd.com

American Spinal Injury Association (ASIA)
2020 Peachtree Road, N.W.
Atlanta, GA 30309
(404) 355-9772

DateAble International
35 Wisconsin Circle
Suite 205
Chevy Chase, MD 20815
(301) 656-8723
e-mail: robert@dateable.org
A dating service by and for the disabled.

Disabled American Veterans
807 Maine Avenue, S.W.
Washington, DC 20024
(202) 554-3501

Disability Rights Education and Defense Fund, Inc.
1633 Q Street, N.W.
Suite 220
Washington, DC 20009
(202) 988-0375
(202) 462-5624 (fax)
West Coast:
2212 Sixth Street
Berkeley, CA 94710
(510) 644-2555
(800) 466-4232 (Voice/TDD)
(510) 841-8845 (fax)

HealthSouth
One HealthSouth Parkway
Birmingham, AL 35243
(800) 765-4772
www.healthsouth.com

HealthSouth Rehabilitation Institute of San Antonio (RIOSA)
9119 Cinnamon Hill
San Antonio, TX 78240
(800) 688-0737

Job Accommodation Network
www.janweb.icdi.wvu.edu
Job information for the disabled.

Microsoft Accessibility and Disabilities Web Site
www.Microsoft.com/enable
Computer accessibility information for the disabled.

National Council on Disability
1331 F Street, N.W.
Suite 1050
Washington, DC 20004
(202) 272-2004
(202) 272-2022 (fax)
www.ncd.gov
A policy advisory board.

National Council on Independent Living (NCIL)
1916 Wilson Boulevard
Suite 209
Arlington, VA 22201
(703) 525-3406
(703) 525-3409 (fax)
(703) 525-4153 (TTY)
e-mail: ncil.tsbbso8.tnet.com
A grassroots advocacy group for the disabled.

National Spinal Cord Injury Association
8300 Colesville Road
Silver Spring, MD 20910
(301) 588-6959
Hotline: (800) 962-9629
e-mail: NSCIA2@aol.com
www.spinalcord.org

New Mobility
An on-line magazine for the spinal cord injured.
www.NewMobility.com
Offers "best of the Web" for the disabled.

SOURCES

Butt, Lester M., and Indira S. Lanig, "Stress Management," *A Practial Guide to Health Promotion After Spinal Cord Injury*, edited by Indira S. Lanig, MD, Theresa M. Chase, MA, RN, Lester M. Butt, PhD, Katy L. Hulse, LCSW, and Kelly M. M. Johnson, RN, Gaithersburg, Maryland: Aspen Publishers, Inc., 1996.

Canedy, Dana, "More Toys are Reflecting Disabled Children's Needs," *The New York Times*, December 25, 1997.

Cardenas, Diana D., Lisa Farrell-Roberts, Marca L. Sipski, and Deborah Rubner, "Management of Gastrointestinal, Genitourinary, and Sexual Function," *Spinal Cord Injury: Clinical Outcomes from the Model Systems*, edited by Samuel L. Stover, MD, Joel A. DeLisa, MD, MS, and Gale G. Whiteneck, PhD, Gaithersburg, Maryland: Aspen Publishers, Inc., 1995.

Cerny, Kay, "Physical Therapy Evaluation, Goal Setting, and Program Planning," *Clinics in Physical Therapy: Spinal Cord Injury*, edited by Hazel V. Atkins, New York: Churchill Livingstone, 1985.

Chase, Theresa M., "Physical Fitness Strategies," *A Practial Guide to Health Promotion After Spinal Cord Injury*, edited by Indira S. Lanig, MD, Theresa M. Chase, MA, RN, Lester M. Butt, PhD, Katy L. Hulse, LCSW, and Kelly M. M. Johnson, RN, Gaithersburg, Maryland: Aspen Publishers, Inc., 1996.

Corbet, Barry, *Options: Spinal Cord Injury and the Future,* Denver: A.B. Hirschfeld Press, 1991.

Corbet, Barry, editor, *National Resource Directory: An Information Guide for Persons with Spinal Cord Injury and Other Physical Disabilities,* Rockville, Maryland: National Spinal Cord Injury Association, 1985.

Edberg, Elwin and Hazel V. Adkins, "Wheelchairs and Cushions," *Clinics in Physical Therapy: Spinal Cord Injury,* edited by Hazel V. Atkins, New York: Churchill Livingstone, 1985.

Farrow, Jeff, "Sexuality Counseling with Clients Who Have Spinal Cord Injuries," *Rehabilitation Counseling Bulletin,* Vol. 33, No. 3, March 1990.

Go, Bette K., Michael J. DeVivo, and J. Scott Richards, "The Epidemiology of Spinal Cord Injury," *Spinal Cord Injury: Clinical Outcomes from the Model Systems,* edited by Samuel L. Stover, MD, Joel A. DeLisa, MD, MS, and Gale G. Whiteneck, PhD, Gaithersburg, Maryland: Aspen Publishers, Inc., 1995.

Grady, Denise, "Spine Researchers Seek Recipe for Regeneration," *The New York Times,* September 30, 1997.

Hammond, Margaret C., M., Robert L. Umlauf, PhD, Brenda Matteson, Sonya Perduta-Fulginiti, *Yes, You Can! A Guide to Self-Care for Persons with Spinal Cord Injury,* Washington, DC: Paralyzed Veterans of America, 1989.

Harari, Danielle, MD, Jerrilyn Quinlan, and Steven A. Stiens, MD, *Constipation and Spinal Cord Injury: A Guide to Symptoms and Treatment,* Washington, DC: Paralyzed Veterans of America.

Hill, Judy P., OTR, *Spinal Cord Injury: A Guide to Functional Outcomes in Occupational Therapy,* Rockville, Maryland: Aspen Publishers, Inc., 1986.

Kiser, Carolyn and Christine Herman, "Nursing Considerations: Skin Care, Bowel and Bladder Training, Autonomic Dysreflexia," *Clinics in Physical Therapy: Spinal Cord Injury,* edited by Hazel V. Atkins, New York: Churchill Livingstone, 1985.

Kuric, Judi, MSC, and Andrea Kaye Hixon, RN, MS, "Clinical Practice Guideline: Autonomic Dysreflexia," Jackson Heights, New York: *American Association of Spinal Cord Injury Nurses,* 1996.

Lanig, Indira S., "Historical Perspectives," *A Practical Guide to Health Promotion After Spinal Cord Injury,* edited by Indira S. Lanig, MD, Theresa M. Chase, MA, RN, Lester M. Butt, PhD, Katy L. Hulse, LCSW, and Kelly M. M. Johnson, RN, Gaithersburg, Maryland: Aspen Publishers, Inc., 1996.

———, "Models, Concepts, and Terminology," *A Practial Guide to Health Promotion After Spinal Cord Injury,* edited by Indira S. Lanig, MD, Theresa M. Chase, MA, RN, Lester M. Butt, PhD, Katy L. Hulse, LCSW, and Kelly M. M. Johnson, RN, Gaithersburg, Maryland: Aspen Publishers, Inc., 1996.

———, "Promoting Nutritional Health," *A Practical Guide to Health Promotion After Spinal Cord Injury,* edited by Indira S. Lanig, MD, Theresa M. Chase, MA, RN, Lester M. Butt, PhD, Katy L. Hulse, LCSW, and Kelly M. M. Johnson, RN, Gaithersburg, Maryland: Aspen Publishers, Inc., 1996.

Maddox, Sam, *Spinal Network,* Boulder, Colorado: Spinal Network and Sam Maddox, 1987.

McCluer, Shirley, MD, and Karen Schmidt, "Syringomyelia," Little Rock, Arkansas: *Arkansas Spinal Cord Commission,* 1996.

Menter, Robert R., and Lesley M. Hudson, "Effects of Age at Injury and the Aging Process," *Spinal Cord Injury: Clinical Outcomes from the Model Systems,* edited by Samuel L. Stover, MD, Joel A. DeLisa, MD, MS, and Gale G. Whiteneck, PhD, Gaithersburg, Maryland: Aspen Publishers, Inc., 1995.

Morgan, Selina Medieta, "A Guide to Choosing Mobility Equipment," *Progress Report,* Fall 1990.

Nixon, Vickie, PT, *Spinal Cord Injury: A Guide to Functional Outcomes in Physical Therapy Management,* Rockville, Maryland: Aspen Publications, Inc., 1985.

O'Hara, Dolores Liszka, RN, *Planning for the Future: A Handbook for Individuals with Spinal Cord Injuries and Their Significant Others,* Pittsburgh: HealthSouth Rehabilitation Hospital, 1995.

Ragnarsson, Kristjan T., Karyl M. Hall, Conal B. Wilmot, and R. Edward Carter, "Management of Pulmonary, Cardiovascular, and Metabolic Conditions after Spinal Cord Injury," *Spinal Cord Injury: Clinical Outcomes from the Model Systems,* edited by Samuel L. Stover, MD, Joel A. DeLisa, MD, MS, and Gale G. Whiteneck, PhD, Gaithersburg, Maryland: Aspen Publishers, Inc., 1995.

Richards, J. Scott, Bette K. Go, Richard D. Rutt, and Patricia B. Lazarus, "The National Spinal Cord Injury Collaborative Database," *Spinal Cord Injury: Clinical Outcomes from the Model Systems,* edited by Samuel L. Stover, MD, Joel A. DeLisa, MD, MS, and Gale G. Whiteneck, PhD, Gaithersburg, Maryland: Aspen Publishers, Inc., 1995.

Schust, Christina S., and Sara Nell Di Lima, *Spinal Cord Injury: Patient Education Manual,* Gaithersburg, Maryland: Aspen Publishers, Inc., 1997.

Senelick, Richard C., MD, and Cathy E. Ryan, MA, CCC-SLP, *Living with Brain Injury: A Guide for Families,* Birmingham: HealthSouth Press, 1998.

———, "Sex and Disability," *San Antonio Medical Gazette,* October 9 and October 15, 1997.

———, "Stroke Rehabilitation: Predicting Functional Outcome," *Outcomes,* Vol. 1, Nos. 17 and 21, 1995.

Somerville, Nancy Jean and Heidi McHugh Pendleton, "Evaluation and Solving Home Access Problems," *Clinics in Physical Therapy: Spinal Cord Injury,* edited by Hazel V. Atkins, New York: Churchill Livingstone, 1985.

Strothcamp, Janeen, "Spinal Cord Injury and Functional Electrical Stimulation," *Progress Report,* Spring 1990.

Stutts, Michael, PhD, Jeffrey S. Kreutzer, PhD, Jeffrey T. Barth, PhD, Thomas Ryan, PhD, Julian Hickman, Catherine W. Devany, and Jennifer H. Marwitz, "Cognitive Impairment in Persons with Recent Spinal Cord Injury: Findings and Implications for Clinical Practice," *Neurorehabilitation,* Vol. 1, No. 3, 1991.

Thomas, J. Paul, "The Model Spinal Cord Injury Concept: Development and Implementation," *Spinal Cord Injury: Clinical Outcomes from the Model Systems,* edited by Samuel L. Stover, MD, Joel A. DeLisa, MD, MS, and Gale G. Whiteneck, PhD, Gaithersburg, Maryland: Aspen Publishers, Inc., 1995.

Weller, Doris J., MSW, and Patricia M. Miller, MSW, "Emotional Reactions of Patient, Family, and Staff in Acute-Care Period of Spinal Cord Injury: Part 1," *Social Work in Health Care,* Vol. 2, No. 41, Summer 1977.

———, "Emotional Reactions of Patient, Family, and Staff in Acute-Care Period of Spinal Cord Injury: Part 2," *Social Work in Health Care,* Vol. 3, No. 1, Fall 1977.

Wetzel, Jane, "Respiratory Evaluation and Treatment," *Clinics in Physical Therapy: Spinal Cord Injury,* edited by Hazel V. Atkins, New York: Churchill Livingstone, 1985.

Yarkony, Gary M., and Allen W. Heinemann, "Pressure Ulcers," *Spinal Cord Injury: Clinical Outcomes from the Model Systems,* edited by Samuel L. Stover, MD, Joel A. DeLisa, MD, MS, and Gale G. Whiteneck, PhD, Gaithersburg, Maryland: Aspen Publishers, Inc., 1995.

————, *Learning and Living After Your Spinal Cord Injury*, Pittsburgh: Harmarville Rehabilitation Center, Inc., 1983.

————, *Standards for Neurological Classification of Spinal Injury Patients*, Atlanta: American Spinal Injury Association.

————, "Fact Sheet #1: Common Questions About Spinal Cord Injury," *National Spinal Cord Injury Association*, Silver Spring, Maryland: National Spinal Cord Injury Association, 1995-1996.

————, "Fact Sheet #2: Spinal Cord Injury Statistical Information," *National Spinal Cord Injury Association*, Silver Spring, Maryland: National Spinal Cord Injury Association, July 1996.

————, "Fact Sheet #4a: Choosing a Spinal Cord Injury Rehabilitation Facility", *National Spinal Cord Injury Association*, Silver Spring, Maryland: National Spinal Cord Injury Association, 1995-1996.

————, "Fact Sheet #5: What's New in Spinal Cord Injury Treatment and Cure Research?" *National Spinal Cord Injury Association*, Silver Spring, Maryland: National Spinal Cord Injury Association,1995-1996.

————, "Fact Sheet #8: Spinal Cord Injury Awareness — Understanding the Importance of Language and Images," *National Spinal Cord Injury Association*, Silver Spring, Maryland: National Spinal Cord Injury Association, 1995-1996.

————, "Fact Sheet #9: Functional Electrical Stimulation, Clinical Applications in Spinal Cord Injury," *National Spinal Cord Injury Association*, Silver Spring, Maryland: National Spinal Cord Injury Association, 1995-1996.

————, "Fact Sheet #10: Male Reproductive Function After Spinal Cord Injury," *National Spinal Cord Injury Association*, Silver Spring, Maryland: National Spinal Cord Injury Association, 1995-1996.

————, "Fact Sheet #17: What is Autonomic Dysreflexia?" *National Spinal Cord Injury Association*, Silver Spring, Maryland: National Spinal Cord Injury Association, 1995-1996.

————, "Fact Sheet #18: Starting a Support Group or a Discussion Group," *National Spinal Cord Injury Association*, Silver Spring, Maryland: National Spinal Cord Injury Association, 1995-1996.

————, "Alcohol Abuse," *RRTC on Aging with Spinal Cord Injury*, Englewood, Colorado: RRTC on Aging with Spinal Cord Injury, 1995.

————, "Am I Ready for a Van?" *RRTC on Aging with Spinal Cord Injury*, Englewood, Colorado: RRTC on Aging with Spinal Cord Injury, 1995.

————, "Aging, SCI and the Battle of the Bulge," *RRTC on Aging with Spinal Cord Injury*, Englewood, Colorado: RRTC on Aging with Spinal Cord Injury, 1995.

————, "Changing or Choosing Your Doctor," *RRTC on Aging with Spinal Cord Injury*, Englewood, Colorado: RRTC on Aging with Spinal Cord Injury, 1995.

————, "Fatigue," *RRTC on Aging with Spinal Cord Injury*, Englewood, Colorado: RRTC on Aging with Spinal Cord Injury, 1995.

————, "Interacting with Your Doctor," *RRTC on Aging with Spinal Cord Injury*,

Englewood, Colorado: RRTC on Aging with Spinal Cord Injury, 1995.

———, "Long Term Caregivers: For Better and For Worse," *RRTC on Aging with Spinal Cord Injury,* Englewood, Colorado: RRTC on Aging with Spinal Cord Injury, 1995.

———, "Personal Care Assistants: How to Find, Hire, and Keep Them," *RRTC on Aging with Spinal Cord Injury,* Englewood, Colorado: RRTC on Aging with Spinal Cord Injury, 1995.

———, "Optimal Health: What It Is and How To Get It," *RRTC on Aging with Spinal Cord Injury,* Englewood, Colorado: RRTC on Aging with Spinal Cord Injury, 1996.

———, "Osteoporosis," *RRTC on Aging with Spinal Cord Injury,* Englewood, Colorado: RRTC on Aging with Spinal Cord Injury, 1995.

———, "Spasticity," *RRTC on Aging with Spinal Cord Injury,* Englewood, Colorado: RRTC on Aging with Spinal Cord Injury, 1995.

———, "Upper Extremity Pain," *RRTC on Aging with Spinal Cord Injury,* Englewood, Colorado: RRTC on Aging with Spinal Cord Injury, 1995.

———, *Sexuality After Your Spinal Cord Injury,* Pittsburgh: Harmarville Rehabilitation Center, Inc., 1985.

———, "Switching to a Power Chair," *RRTC on Aging with Spinal Cord Injury,* Englewood, Colorado: RRTC on Aging with Spinal Cord Injury, 1996.

INDEX

About the Authors

RICHARD C. SENELICK, MD, is the Medical Director at the HealthSouth Rehabilitation Institute of San Antonio (RIOSA). He also serves as Program Director of its Brain Injury program. A native of Illinois, Dr. Senelick completed his undergraduate and medical school training at the University of Illinois in Chicago. A neurologist who specializes in neurorehabilitation, he subsequently completed his neurology training at the University of Utah in Salt Lake City. Dr. Senelick has authored numerous publications, including co-authoring *Living with Brain Injury: A Guide for Families* and *Living with Stroke: A Guide for Families*. The Editor in Chief of HealthSouth Press, Dr. Senelick is also a member of the National Stroke Association Rehabilitation Advisory Board.

KARLA DOUGHERTY has written 29 books, many of them in the medical field. She is a co-author of *Living with Stroke: A Guide for Families,* and has collaborated with Dr. Senelick on several other titles as well. She is the Senior Writer for HealthSouth Press. Ms. Dougherty is also a member of the Author's Guild and the American Medical Writers Association. She lives in New Jersey.

"Getting People Back" - The HEALTHSOUTH Rehabilitation Series

Getting people back... to work... to play... to living. It has been the HEALTHSOUTH commitment since we first started taking care of people with disabilities and injuries. Now HEALTHSOUTH Press continues this tradition with "Getting People Back" - The HEALTHSOUTH Rehabilitation Series.

These books are specifically designed for people who need up-to-date, authoritative, and easy-to-access knowledge about their problems. In a user-friendly, simple manner, these books help educate patients and their families.

HEALTHSOUTH Press will continue its partnership with a broad base of communities by donating profits to charity through the HEALTHSOUTH Foundation.

Through knowledge and education comes empowerment and the ability to do more than just "live" with a disability. These books provide the opportunity to exceed expectations and get people back.

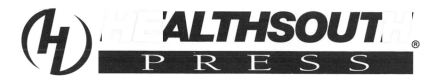

HEALTHSOUTH PRESS

The HEALTHSOUTH Press Library is dedicated to helping people get back to their lives after trauma, an accident or an illness. Our books demonstrate, in compassionate yet authoritative terms, how you can overcome your disability and live a full, rich life.

Utilizing the experience and up-to-the-minute technology of our vast network of rehabilitation hospitals and skilled physicians, therapists and health professionals, HEALTHSOUTH Press promises to show you a new and better way to adjust to a new life. Our books provide hope. Not false hope, but possible, viable and very real hope.

If you would like to order additional copies of *The Spinal Cord Injury Handbook for Patients and Their Families*, please mail the coupon below to: HEALTHSOUTH Press, 9119 Cinnamon Hill, San Antonio, TX 78240. You can also visit our Web site at www.healthsouth.com

We are also pleased to offer copies of *Living with Brain Injury: A Guide for Families* at $8.95 each ($2 off the list price of $10.95). Please include $2.50 for postage and handling.

❏ Enclosed is my check/money order made payable to HEALTHSOUTH Press for *Living with Brain Injury: A Guide for Families* at $12.95, plus shipping and handling (for a total of $11.45).

❏ Enclosed is my check/money order made payable to HEALTHSOUTH Press for *The Spinal Cord Injury Handbook for Patients and Their Families* at $12.95 each, plus shipping and handling (for a total of $15.45).

(If you would like more than one copy of either title, please write in the quantity and title below.

Name_____

Title_____

Address_____

City/State/Zip_____

Phone_____

I'd like_____additional copies of_____
　　　(# of books)　　　　　　　　　　　　　　　　　(titles of books)

For additional information, please call 800 688-0737.